IBD

SELF-MANAGEMENT

IBD
SELF-MANAGEMENT

THE AGA GUIDE TO CROHN'S DISEASE AND ULCERATIVE COLITIS

Sunanda V. Kane, MD, MSPH

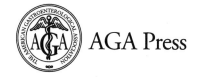 AGA Press

IBD Self-Management
The AGA Guide to Crohn's Disease and Ulcerative Colitis

AGA Institute Publications Committee

Michael Camilleri, MD, AGAF, Chair

Damian H. Augustyn, MD, AGAF   Marshall H. Montrose, PhD
Fred S. Gorelick, MD   Cindy Yoshida, MD, AGAF

AGA Press Advisory Board

Colin W. Howden, MD, AGAF, Chair   Lawrence J. Brandt, MD, AGAF
Melinda Dennis, MS, RD   Benjamin D. Gold, MD
Steven Flamm, MD   Monica Jarrett, PhD, RN
David C. Metz, MD, AGAF   Melissa Palmer, MD
Amy Shaheen, MD   Helen M. Shields, MD, AGAF

AGA Press

Christine B. Charlip	*Division Director of Publications*
Sherrye Landrum	*Book Editor*
Sarah Williamson	*Medical Illustrator*
Studio Grafik	*Cover Design*
Circle Graphics, Inc.	*Page Design and Composition*
McNaughton & Gunn, Inc.	*Printing*

Disclaimer

This publication provides accurate information on the subject matter covered. The publisher is not providing legal, medical, or other professional services. Reference herein to any specific commercial products, procedures, or services by trade name, trademark, manufacturer, or otherwise does not constitute or imply endorsement, recommendation, or favored status by the AGA Institute. The views and opinions of the author(s) expressed in this publication do not necessarily state or reflect those of the AGA Institute, and they shall not be used to advertise or endorse a product.

Printed in the United States of America

13 12 11 10   1 2 3 4 5 6

ISBN 978-1-60356-005-4

Library of Congress Control Number: 2009912969

For additional copies or information on licensing or translating this content, please contact:

AGA Press
4930 Del Ray Avenue
Bethesda, MD 20814-2513
www.gastro.org/publications

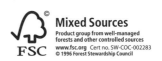

Mixed Sources
Product group from well-managed forests and other controlled sources
www.fsc.org   Cert no. SW-COC-002283
© 1996 Forest Stewardship Council

To my father, who pushed me incessantly because he knew I could accomplish great things if I just put my mind to it.

To Stephen Hanauer, MD, the best role model a young physician could ever have. He taught me the art of caring for patients, and I will always be indebted to him.

To my husband, who was so exquisitely patient, caring, and supportive while I spent even less time with him than usual to write this book.

Contents

11 Taking Charge of Your Lifestyle 177

Foreword

Whether you are newly diagnosed with Crohn's disease or ulcerative colitis or have been living with inflammatory bowel disease (IBD) for many years, having credible and accurate information is crucial to your health. But finding the right resource on IBD can be a daunting task. It's easy to feel overwhelmed weeding through the sea of information, whether on the Internet or in the vast array of scientific research and the many books.

The Crohn's & Colitis Foundation of America (CCFA) hears from hundreds of people daily who are searching for information on how to best manage and cope with their IBD. It is our priority to connect people with accurate information that will arm them with the knowledge and power they need to improve their quality of life and take control of their disease. It is also our priority to ensure that the resources we are recommending are unbiased and balanced. CCFA has enthusiastically added *IBD Self-Management: The AGA Guide to Crohn's Disease and Ulcerative Colitis* by Dr. Sunanda V. Kane to our vast resource library. This valuable guide can be shared with anyone who is living with, or knows someone with, IBD. Easy to read and written in a supportive voice, it provides a thorough overview on everything you need to know about IBD and answers core questions about Crohn's disease and ulcerative colitis. It is filled with stories that bring to life the diverse experiences that many people can face because of IBD.

You are in good hands as you read what Dr. Kane shares with you. I have had the pleasure of closely collaborating with her as she has served as a dedicated advisor and volunteer for the CCFA. Her wisdom and expertise have helped to shape many of the resources that we provide to people living with IBD. Dr. Kane's honest approach, coupled with her dedication and sensitivity to people's needs, is intrinsic throughout this book. We are lucky to have Dr. Kane, someone who is committed to making a positive impact on the lives of all who are affected by IBD, working with the CCFA and sharing her wisdom with all who read this book.

We are grateful that Dr. Kane and the American Gastroenterological Association have created this unique and valuable resource for all of those living with and affected by IBD.

Kimberly Frederick
Vice President, Patient & Professional Services
The Crohn's & Colitis Foundation of America

Preface

Writing *IBD Self-Management* was a true labor of love. It is what I would want to teach you if you were a patient newly diagnosed with inflammatory bowel disease (IBD) who was sitting in my office. Although I tried to cover as many topics as I could, because the field of IBD is changing so quickly, it would be impossible to be absolutely complete. Also, your IBD is a personal disease: you are a little bit different in how it affects you and what you need to do to live successfully with it. So, although this book covers the topics that are of concern to most of the patients that I meet—and some you may not have even thought of or experienced—you will need to look at it through the lens of your own goals and abilities to get the most out of this information.

As I go through with you, in detail, the challenges of living with IBD, please do not consider me a voice of "doom and gloom." It's just the opposite. The more you understand about IBD, the more insight you will have into your options and the better you will be able to help yourself. So many of my patients lead productive, happy, and well-adjusted lives, and the prognosis of both ulcerative colitis and Crohn's disease has become so much brighter over the past decade. We've developed better medical therapies that permit healing and surgical techniques that spare the bowel and have more cosmetically appealing outcomes. I feel very fortunate to have such an active role in a field that is rapidly improving the lives of people who have IBD.

Nutrition is probably the most important topic for most patients, and certainly the one in which I field the greatest number of questions. Therefore, it was appropriate to have some more input. I turned to Susan Hopson, RD, who was a valued member of the Gastroenterology Clinic at the University of Chicago when I was on faculty there and who helped us quite a bit with our patients and their individual nutritional needs. Many thanks to Sue for her major contributions to Chapter 10.

The information in this book is based on clinical research, controlled trials, and personal experience or communications with trusted colleagues in the field. The Mayo Clinic does not hold any responsibility for the contents of this book; their only link to this book is my affiliation with the institution.

I hope that this book informs and enables you. I asked many patients what they would like to have in a book about their disease, and I listened. *IBD Self-Management: The AGA Guide to Crohn's Disease and Ulcerative Colitis* is for all of them, as well as for the patients I may never meet but may be able to help.

Sunanda V. Kane, MD, MSPH
Mayo Clinic
Rochester, Minnesota

Acknowledgments

It is important that I thank several people who took time out of their very busy schedules to review this book for its content. David T. Rubin, MD; Lawrence J. Brandt, MD, AGAF; Melissa Palmer, MD; David I. Weinberg, MD; and Corey A. Siegel, MD, each offered invaluable suggestions that strengthened the book and its message. The staff at the Crohn's & Colitis Foundation of America also reviewed the book, and I appreciate their input.

Because I do not care for many pediatric patients, I obtained the input and counsel of Marci Reiss, LCSW, a dedicated social worker whose purpose is to help those families struggling to make sense of their lives when a child is affected. She kindly offered to share with the readers some of her sage advice for parents who have children with IBD (see Chapter 12). She is also president of the IBD Support Foundation, a worthy organization that helps patients with ulcerative colitis or Crohn's disease and their families through support groups and counseling programs.

1

Why IBD?
Why Me?

L ife is hard for Joanna. She has to be aware at all times of the
location of a bathroom and is in constant fear of an accident.
This has put a big dent in her social life, and she often turns down invitations. Joanna's joints hurt, and she is much more fatigued than she
thinks a 27-year-old should be.

Does this sound like you? I hope not. But perhaps you react this way
when your inflammatory bowel disease (IBD) is active or undertreated.
IBD is a lifelong condition, but it does not have to be "an illness." What's
sad about Joanna is that she has become angry, complacent, and dis-
illusioned about her situation. She dwells on the idea that she can't be
cured. Once you give up, nothing is going to help you. Joanna has
repeatedly refused referrals to a medical center that specializes in treating IBD, despite the urging of her doctors. She puts faith in the doctors
she has always gone to and expects them to know everything. She stops

her medicines without telling anyone, for one reason or another. She relies on the local hospital emergency room when she finds herself in need of urgent care rather than keeping her appointments. She reads Internet sites that scare her more than educate her and takes advice from well-meaning but uneducated friends, neighbors, and coworkers. She won't take the vitamins her doctors suggest even though she knows she is iron deficient. She often asks, "Why me?"

It's obvious to everyone but Joanna that she won't help herself. We doctors understand that some people can't be helped, but some people *won't* be helped. Although there is no cure for IBD yet, we have ways to treat it that are improving every day. But any physician can only do so much. The plain truth is that, when you have IBD, how you fare is your choice. Please believe that there is a path to making peace and finding health when you live with IBD. You can find your own way by taking control of your body and your disease and learning all you can about responsible things you can do to help yourself. This book has reliable information on how to live your best life. Having met and cared for thousands of people facing IBD, I am convinced that you have the ability to succeed at living with and managing your IBD.

Gastrointestinal Anatomy

To self-manage your IBD, it will help to understand the anatomy of the gastrointestinal (GI) tract (Figure 1). It starts in the mouth and consists of the esophagus; stomach; small intestine, which is divided up into three sections: duodenum, jejunum, and ileum; colon (large intestine or bowel); rectum; and anus. The terminal ileum is the last few inches of the ileum.

We generally divide the colon into three parts: the rectum, the left side, and the right side (Figure 2). Although it is physically attached to the colon, the rectum is supplied by a different network of nerves and blood vessels than the rest of the colon and so is considered its own section. The left side is made up of the sigmoid and descending colon, and sometimes part of the transverse colon. The right side is the top half of

FIGURE 1. The Gastrointestinal Tract

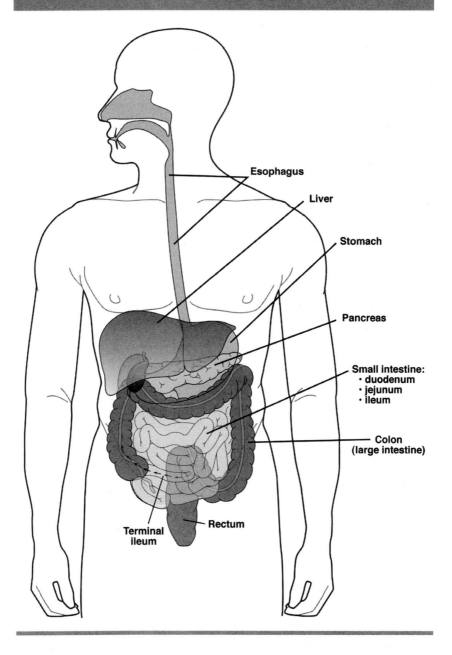

FIGURE 2. Colon Anatomy

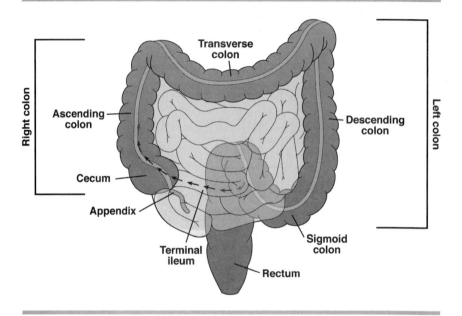

---

the transverse colon, ascending colon, and cecum. The appendix hangs from the cecum.

The colon is made up of multiple layers. The innermost layer of cells, called the *mucosa,* works to absorb water from stool. This is the main function of the colon: to absorb water from waste material sent from the small intestine and to package it for removal from the body. The mucosa is seen with the endoscope and is what is sampled during a biopsy. The other layers, moving from the inside to the outside of the colon, are connective tissue, muscle, and an outer lining that contains nerve cells.

In addition to these layers, there are glands in the colon, rectum, and anal canal that produce mucus. Mucus helps lubricate stool so that it slides out more readily when you are pushing during a bowel movement. Normally, mucus stays within the rectum and you do not see it. It gets reabsorbed and new mucus is produced. When there is inflammation or irritation, these glands become more active and more mucus is produced. When you have a lot of diarrhea, mucus can come out with the stool rather than stay within the rectum. Mucus in the stool is often a sign of inflammation but may occur in other conditions such as irritable bowel syndrome (see page 7).

What Is Inflammation?

Inflammation is the reaction of the body to anything foreign. It is a natural process that is essential for health. "Foreign" can be practically anything—from a splinter in the finger to the poison in a bee sting or bacteria in tainted tuna salad. The natural reaction of the body to this foreign thing is to attack it and get rid of it, either by engulfing and digesting it or by destroying it. We experience inflammation as swelling, redness, warmth, and pain, all caused by proteins that are produced during the attack-and-destroy process.

Sometimes the body is tricked into thinking that some portion or product of the body is foreign, and then it attacks itself. This is what we call an *autoimmune disease.* There are many examples of autoimmune diseases, like lupus, type 1 diabetes, and inflammatory bowel disease.

Inflammatory Bowel Disease Defined

IBD is characteristically a lifelong (chronic) condition in which there is inflammation of the lining of the gastrointestinal tract for no apparent reason. The inflammation might be located just in one part of the digestive tract, for example, in the large intestine (colon), but it can appear anywhere along the digestive tract, from the mouth to the anus.

IBD occurs as two major types and two rare types. Ulcerative colitis (Chapter 2) and Crohn's disease (Chapter 3) are the two diseases that most people recognize because they are the most common. Chapter 4 takes a look at two other less common types of IBD.

More than 1 million Americans have IBD, and right now this is equally split between Crohn's disease and ulcerative colitis. However, this balance is likely to change because the number of new cases of Crohn's disease is on the rise, although the reason behind this trend is not entirely clear. Each year, approximately 10 people per 100,000 are diagnosed with ulcerative colitis and 16 people per 100,000 are diagnosed with Crohn's disease.[1]

It's most common to develop IBD between the ages of 15 and 35. However, children as young as 3 years old have been diagnosed. There is a second peak of diagnosis between ages 50 and 55. IBD occurs equally in men and women.[2] In Americans, it tends to occur more often in Caucasians, particularly of Jewish descent. However, more African-Americans and Latinos are being diagnosed each year. In truth, there are no longer "typical" patients in terms of ethnicity. People living in all parts of the United States get IBD, so there are no geographical differences here. Globally, IBD tends to occur in industrialized nations rather than developing countries and appears to be associated with better sanitation, for reasons that aren't understood.[3]

Were You Misdiagnosed?

It's possible. Many symptoms of Crohn's disease and ulcerative colitis mimic other conditions. For instance, short-term inflammation in the gut can be caused by infection with bacteria, viruses, or parasites. Taking medications like ibuprofen can cause symptoms of colitis, such as pain, cramping, and diarrhea, that might be mistaken for IBD. Sometimes blood tests will suggest IBD without other supporting information. (There is more about correct diagnosis in Chapters 2 and 3.) In fact, there are a multitude of conditions that can act like IBD or look like IBD on an X-ray or colonoscopy. In some individuals, IBD is very hard to find at first, and it is not until you have spent some time living with the symptoms that it becomes apparent that chronic inflammation is occurring.

This was the case with Miriam, a 72-year-old woman with bad arthritis of the knees. She was referred to me for "unresolving colitis." Miriam, who takes ibuprofen on a regular basis for her knee pain, developed blood in her stools and was worried that she had colon cancer. A colonoscopy revealed inflammation of her colon, and the samples of the colon lining (biopsies) also seemed to indicate inflammation. Believing that Miriam had ulcerative colitis, the doctor started her on medications for that, but she continued to bleed. Despite even stronger medications, her symptoms continued. That's when Miriam was referred to me for a second opinion. I carefully reviewed her biopsies under the microscope. It turned out that Miriam had acute, not chronic, inflammation, much more consistent with damage from taking ibuprofen rather than a chronic condition like ulcerative colitis. She discontinued ulcerative colitis medications, and we discussed how she could try physical therapy to treat her knees rather than high doses of ibuprofen. After a couple of weeks off ibuprofen, Miriam's bleeding stopped and her colon returned to normal.

It's easy to mix up IBD and irritable bowel syndrome (IBS).[4] They occur in the same area of the body, and they often share similar symptoms, such as pain and diarrhea. But a thorough medical exam with diagnostic testing can make the distinction between IBD and IBS.

IBS is estimated to occur in 15% of the U.S. population or about 50 million people. Although the cause of IBS is not completely understood, it appears that IBS occurs when there are problems with the nerves that control gut function.[5] You may hear that a diagnosis of IBS is one of exclusion. This is because there are no specific tests for IBS; instead, the diagnosis is made using specific symptom criteria.[6] Therefore, other possible causes are excluded before coming to the conclusion that what is wrong is most likely IBS. With IBS, there is no active inflammation of the gastrointestinal tract, so there are no bouts of bleeding or fevers that are common with IBD. In IBD, there is chronic inflammation that sometimes flares up. The damage that occurs with IBD can be serious and requires treatment, whereas the symptoms of IBS can go away without treatment. Some people with IBS struggle with almost constant digestive issues. Although this can be quite disruptive, they are not life-threatening.

Keep in mind that having IBD does not make you immune to IBS. Studies suggest that as many as half of the people diagnosed with Crohn's disease have IBS, and a third of patients with ulcerative colitis have IBS as well.[7]

Because you have received a diagnosis of IBD, you owe yourself a visit to a doctor who is a specialist in IBD. All gastroenterologists receive training in IBD, but some take a special interest in its diagnosis and management, just as others might specialize in the pancreas or liver. You may like and respect your own doctor, but it never hurts to meet with someone really up-to-date on IBD to review your current health and care plan. After all, we are talking about a lifelong disease, and the right diagnosis and treatment plan ultimately make for the best outcomes. If you are worried about creating hard feelings, be sure to tell your doctor up front that you like and trust him or her and just want to include the viewpoint of an expert eye. IBD experts can be found in small private practices as well as large university medical centers. The Crohn's & Colitis Foundation of America is an excellent source of information and can help you find a physician who is a member of that organization and treats more people with IBD than perhaps other physicians in your community.

Despite what you may think, the future remains very bright for people with IBD. Yes, we want a cure and are actively working toward it. But in the meantime, there are ways to manage the disease and minimize symptoms and side effects, including developments in surgical techniques that will help as well.

The Clues about Cause

There are no simple answers to the question of why you developed IBD. The reality is that we don't know why you got ulcerative colitis or Crohn's disease. Many popular theories have been proposed over the years that have not panned out, such as eating refined sugar, drinking pasteurized milk, refrigerating foodstuffs, using toothpaste, and receiving the measles vaccine, just to name a few. It's just not that simple. Research scientists believe that a combination of an individual's genetics and immune system plus environment somehow come together like the "perfect storm" to result in IBD. Let's look at each of these factors.

Genetics

So far, studying genes associated with IBD has failed to reveal whether they have a role in the disease. IBD is different from disorders such as sickle cell disease or cystic fibrosis, in which a single gene is responsible for a very specific mutation that leads to disease. For a time, it seemed that the NOD2 gene might be responsible for causing Crohn's disease. This was an extremely exciting discovery by two different investigators using two different techniques at the same time. The NOD2 gene resembles a gene found in plants that helps them resist bacterial infestation and the disease that results.[8] In humans, the function of the gene is to help the body handle specific kinds of bacteria. A mutation of this gene leads to impaired handling of these bacteria. It may be that the inability to handle bacteria, along with other factors that we have yet to fully understand, may lead to the final pathway of IBD. This is intriguing because one of the theories as to the cause of Crohn's disease is by infection with a mycobacterium species (see page 12).

Scientists are actively studying other genes that are associated with, but not a direct cause of, either Crohn's disease or ulcerative colitis: IL23R, IRGM, ATG16L1, and TLR2, 3, 4, 5, 6, and 9. These genes, when mutated or "defective," show up more often in patients with IBD. For instance, the IRGM and ATG16L1 genes play a role in *autophagy,* which is the body's way of dealing with old and "broken" cells and a process that leads, eventually, to death. When the body is unable to correctly choose which cells should be alive and allowed to function and which need to be broken down and disposed of, it can lead to disease.

Most people who develop IBD do not necessarily have one or all of these defective genes. Only 8% to 17% of those diagnosed with Crohn's disease show evidence of having two abnormal NOD2 genes; 27% to 32% have one abnormal NOD2 gene.[9] Furthermore, if you happen to carry one of these defective genes, you are not guaranteed to develop IBD. On the other hand, not having them does not make you immune to

IBD. So, it is not particularly helpful to test for the presence of any of the genes associated with IBD.

A patient will often ask me about his or her chances of getting Crohn's or ulcerative colitis if a family member has it. Although this may not be true for you, most people with IBD do not have a family member known to have the disease. People will also ask about the possibility of "passing it along" to children. But IBD is not a genetic disorder in the strictest sense. Factors other than genetics are involved in development of the disease.

Here are a few facts about heredity and IBD:

- Thirty percent of those diagnosed have a family history of IBD.
- The chance of getting IBD if a family member has it is greatest if it is a first-degree relative (a parent or sibling), but your risk is still higher than the normal population if the relative is second degree, like a cousin.
- The chance of passing IBD to your child is roughly 3% to 7%.
- If both parents have IBD, the chance of their child developing IBD increases to 45%. However, there is no specific recommendation that couples who both have IBD be counseled about having children, because IBD is not a genetic disease like sickle cell anemia or cystic fibrosis, where counseling is very common.

Immune System

The immune system, which keeps our bodies healthy by resisting foreign invaders, seems to play a starring role in IBD. The immune system is made of cells that act depending on what the body needs to do to defend itself. Sometimes one of the protective things the body needs is inflammation. Perhaps IBD occurs when the immune system overreacts to an infection or injury and keeps producing proteins that end up causing inflammation in your gastrointestinal tract. It may help you understand what is happening in your own body if you look at how the immune system works. We will consider both "innate" immunity and "humoral" immunity.

Some investigators believe that a defect in innate immunity causes IBD. Innate immunity is created by those blood cells that respond within the first minute to an injury or infection, like a burn or insect bite. These cells are produced by the bone marrow.

Studies of treatments that interact with bone marrow show some promise for treating IBD in certain patients. The treatments involve growth hormone, proteins that stimulate bone marrow production of blood cells involved in innate immunity, and stem cell transplants.[10–12] These treatments can alter innate immunity and, perhaps, return it to normal functioning. So far, studies done in humans have been small. Because the long-term effects of manipulating the immune system in this manner are not known and it has the potential to stimulate the growth of tumors, research has slowed in this area.

The second line of defense in the immune system is called *humoral immunity,* which involves the cells that are called into action 24 hours after an "insult," like an injury or infection. An example of humoral immunity are the antibodies your body makes after you receive a vaccination or after you have an infection. Another type of humoral immunity involves the cells that form scar tissue to help heal wounds.

Some researchers believe that IBD is the result of an "overreaction" by humoral immunity. The cells involved in humoral immunity make certain products such as proteins to fight infection or create scar tissue. Therapies we currently use to treat IBD mainly target the humoral immune system and get it to stop producing the specific proteins that are found in blood and tissues of people with IBD.

Tumor necrosis factor (TNF), one of the humoral immune system proteins, is an important target of therapy. TNF has become famous. It was first discovered in the blood of rats that had been bred to develop large cancers to study the effects of different chemotherapies. That's why the name has the word "tumor" in it. It was not until much later that scientists figured out that TNF was not made by cancer cells but is produced by the body as part of a normal response to an insult. Because it is very powerful in causing inflammation, blocking the action of TNF is a successful therapy for many people with IBD, as well as other inflammatory conditions. However, we don't want to completely shut down

TNF action, because it assists in fighting off what the body sees as foreign and helping save our lives from infections.

What is fascinating is that the terminal ileum (the narrow end of the small intestine, just before the colon) is where most of the immune activity for the gut happens, and this is the area most likely to be involved in Crohn's disease. The lymph system works with the immune system in resisting and healing disease. There is lymphatic tissue throughout the GI tract but most is at the end of the small intestine.

Environment

There are two different environments, the one around us and the one within us. The environment around us is essentially the air we breathe and what we eat and drink. For example, we know that cigarette smokers are much more likely to develop Crohn's disease than nonsmokers and that cigarette smoking makes Crohn's disease worse.[13] Our food or water may contain factors that cause illness. Many people have food allergies. For them, exposure to a nutrient like the lactose in milk causes inflammation of the gastrointestinal tract, which results in cramping, bloating, and diarrhea.

Food may contain organisms, such as bacteria, that upset the natural balance of bacteria in our gut. Taking antibiotics may also disrupt the natural bacterial balance of the gut. An infection with certain organisms can lead to chronic inflammation of the gut and make IBD worse. On the other hand, taking in more of the naturally occurring intestinal bacteria by drinking or eating probiotics appears to be helpful for some people with or without IBD. There is more information about this in Chapter 6.

The idea that a particular species of mycobacteria—*Mycobacterium avium* subspecies *paratuberculosis* (MAP)—is the cause of Crohn's disease is under active investigation.[14] Researchers have been able to culture this bacterium from the tissue of some patients with Crohn's disease. It is found mainly in livestock and causes a condition in dairy cows that looks like Crohn's disease. It is thought that MAP can be spread to humans via unpasteurized milk and perhaps through the air. In small studies, a course of antibiotics against MAP has successfully treated Crohn's symptoms in some individuals.[15] However, no cause-and-effect relationship has been proven. To prove that MAP is the cause of Crohn's disease,

- MAP would need to be present in every person with Crohn's
- treatment of MAP would need to cure Crohn's completely
- scientists would need to be able to cause Crohn's if they infected someone with MAP

Obviously, we won't expose healthy people to MAP to see if they develop Crohn's disease. As tempting as it is to blame a single agent, and as much as I would like to believe it, there is not enough strong evidence to be able to say that MAP causes Crohn's disease. For now, I continue to believe that three important factors—your genetics, immune system, and environment—interact to cause Crohn's and other forms of IBD. And lacking knowledge of the exact cause, the only advice I can give about how to avoid or prevent IBD is to encourage those of you with a family history of Crohn's disease not to smoke.

Dealing with Your Feelings

Quality of life studies have shown that most people with IBD feel about the same as those in the healthy population.[16] The exception to this is when the disease is flaring and you are dealing with a bout of inflammation. The unpredictability of disease symptoms and embarrassing problems like urgency, gas, and fecal incontinence definitely add to the burden of having IBD. So it's not surprising that studies suggest that more people with IBD have signs and symptoms of depression than the rest of the population.[17] The unfortunate fact is that depression often goes undiagnosed or untreated.

The Predictable Steps

The five stages of grief as described by Elizabeth Kübler-Ross are very applicable to IBD.[18] Consider each of them on your own terms and in the context of where you are now. Doing this may help you appreciate what you are feeling, and that's the first step you need to take to self-manage your IBD.

Denial. A typical response I hear to the news that someone has IBD is, "This can't be Crohn's disease; it must be an infection or parasite." You may visit several different doctors and hear the same thing. I encourage people to get a second opinion, especially from an institution that has a special interest or strength in IBD. It is when you have been to your fourth doctor and heard the same thing that it is time to accept the diagnosis and move on.

From those who've been diagnosed for some time, I commonly hear, "I don't think this is a flare. It is probably just something I ate or the flu." You have to listen to your body and really think about whether your symptoms are consistent with a flare—but you just don't want to believe it—or whether you really have caught the flu that was going around the community or office. The longer you deny active symptoms, the more likely you are to need more aggressive therapy to deal with their effects. It is better to face reality and be proactive than dawdle and procrastinate and potentially create more problems for yourself.

Anger. "Why me? I didn't deserve this!" Of course you didn't, but being angry does not solve anything nor is it a productive use of your time and energy. I tell my patients that everyone has a handicap but some just hide it better than others. We all think that other people are perfect or have it all together, but it is not true. The sooner you can stop being angry at yourself or the world, the sooner you can move on toward positive behaviors.

Bargaining. "If I just eat better and give up smoking, this will all go away." I hear patients say that all the time. I wish it were true. Changing your diet can help your symptoms and your overall health (see Chapter 10) but it won't stop the inflammatory process. Making changes that benefit you is absolutely a great response but it won't make the IBD go away.

Depression. People with IBD have a higher rate of depression than found in the healthy population, and a lot of it can go undiagnosed and/or untreated.[17] Being unable to work, socialize, or eat what you want or having constant pain all can lead to either a situational depression or prolonged depressive state. No one would necessarily blame you but *not* doing anything about it is counterproductive. Sometimes treating the depression is *more* important than treating the underlying disease.

Some antidepressants have potential side effects that can work to our advantage. Some actually stimulate the appetite, and others have a constipating effect. There is no longer a stigma about being on an antidepressant, nor is it viewed as a "crutch" or a weakness on your part if you need something to help with your mood. What can become addictive are some of the medications used for anxiety, which should be considered short-term therapy.

Acceptance. The last stage of the grieving process is acceptance. This is when you can move on and take the actions that help you get better. Sometimes you will try things that don't work, but a positive attitude about your condition makes it easier to have open discussions with your health care providers about your concerns and issues. There are also good data to suggest that patients with positive attitudes respond better to therapies and overall have better outcomes.

Telling Others

Explaining your IBD to others can be extremely difficult and traumatic. And depending on whom you are trying to tell, the consequences can feel devastating. It's tricky when, on the outside, you look perfectly normal, but you are actually feeling quite terrible. It can be embarrassing to have to rush to the restroom throughout the day or try to explain why you cannot accept a dinner invitation because of how you need to eat.

Family members. It is important to share your news about having IBD with family members because of the genetic element. Having a family member with IBD makes someone more at risk for it also. It may be that your family will be relieved when you tell them; they may have noticed long before you did that there was something wrong. Explain that while there may be an increased risk, this is not an infectious disease, and they will not "catch it" from you.

Friends. It may be that your friends also noticed signs that you weren't well before you did, and if they are really friends, they will be supportive in your disclosure. Not telling them may lead to hard feelings and misunderstandings if you continually decline invitations or leave early from events. They may think that you don't want to spend time with them! You will be surprised how many people, upon learning that you have ulcerative colitis or Crohn's disease, will say "Boy, I know so and so with it, too," or even more shocking, "I have it, too, and never told anyone."

Potential partners. Dating can be such a stressful activity, and the timing of when to tell someone you are dating that you have ulcerative colitis or Crohn's can be so tough. Part of how a potential partner may take the news is how you met—were you set up by friends who maybe knew of your condition, was this a match from an online source or a perhaps the doctor's office where you get care? Sometimes the situation arises before you want it to, like having to run for a washroom when you weren't prepared. That may actually be the perfect time, as you can use that event as the springboard to a conversation regarding your diagnosis.

The timing for such a conversation should not necessarily be on the first date, but neither do you want to wait so long that you feel like you have wasted invested time with someone who turns out to be unaccepting of your condition. A lot of it depends on your personality, how open you are with others, and how accepting you are of others' shortcomings. A lot of people can't hide their "imperfections" or handicaps, like those in wheelchairs or with disfiguring maladies. They have to be up front when meeting new people. Remember that no one is perfect, no matter how it appears. We all face challenges, and yours is IBD.

Examples I have heard from my patients include a discussion around the third or fourth date that starts off, "Did you wonder why I stay away from the salad bar when we go out to eat? Well . . ." or, "It may seem like I spend a lot more time in the washroom than some of your other friends. It is not because I am vain, but . . ."

Coworkers, boss, employer. This is another tough situation. On the one hand, you don't want people to feel sorry for you or discriminate against you because of your condition. On the other hand, you want people to understand and be somewhat more forgiving if you are having a bad day, week, or even month. Your health care provider may be able to help in this instance, with a letter to your employer or boss that will pave the way for certain accommodations to be made for you, like having your desk near a washroom or limiting how much weight you are required to lift. In return, however, you have to be willing to meet people half-way and perform your duties to the best of your abilities so that no one begrudges you "special favors." Maybe you don't want special favors, but having someone at work who understands your situation will be helpful on those days when you can't perform at your best.

Eating Disorders

I want to add a special note about eating disorders. There are times when people with Crohn's disease are diagnosed inappropriately with an eating disorder because their diets are so limited (whether that is their choice or disease induced). There are times, however, when I've seen individuals take it upon themselves to limit what they eat so severely that indeed they could be classified as anorexics because of their aversion to food. Anorexia is a condition that can also go undiagnosed, as many health care providers assume that your Crohn's is keeping you underweight and malnourished. You may also get misdiagnosed as bulimic if it's noticed that you are in the bathroom all the time after a meal, whether to have a bowel movement or vomit. That is why it is important to share your diagnosis with the people who spend the most time around you.

Medical Definitions Used in Ulcerative Colitis and Crohn's Disease

Acute inflammation: inflammation present for less than 6 weeks.

Anus: the end of the colon, which is made up of muscular tissue that, when healthy, controls the exit of stool and air.

Chronic inflammation: inflammation present for longer than 6 weeks.

Colitis: inflammation of the colon. Colitis can be caused by infection, drugs, or a lack of blood flow to the colon. Many people use the word "colitis" when referring to ulcerative colitis, which can be confusing because there are many kinds of colitis, including Crohn's colitis.

Colon: large intestine. Depending on your body size, your colon is about 3–4 feet in length. The primary job of the colon is to absorb water from waste material so the fluid can be used by the rest of the body.

Constipation: fewer than two stools per week. Many patients will complain of constipation when what they really mean is that they have to strain to evacuate or that their stools are very hard.

Diarrhea: the medical definition is when there is more than 200 grams of stool output per 24-hour period. This is about 7 ounces. Having loose or frequent stools does *not* necessarily mean that you have true diarrhea.

Enteritis: inflammation of the small intestine.

Fissure: a break in the tissue around the anal canal.

Fistula: an abnormal connection or tunnel between two body parts.

Ileitis: inflammation of the ileum, the last part of the small intestine.

Inflammation: swelling of tissues beyond normal, which is the body's way of fighting off something foreign. Inflammation can be seen in a tissue biopsy under the microscope. In a tissue biopsy, the shape of the intestinal cells is "warped": instead of cells being nicely rounded in shape, the cells are distorted into oblong shapes.

–itis (suffix): inflammation.

Mucosa: the inner lining of the intestine.

Stenosis: abnormal narrowing of the bowel due to scar tissue, not inflammation.

Stricture: a narrowing of the small or large intestine, most likely due to long-standing inflammation and scar tissue.

Transmural: occurring through the entire width of the intestine wall.

Ulcer: an area of damaged tissue, and in IBD, breakdown of the lining of the intestine.

Ulcerative: inflammation that has damaged the inside of the inner lining of the colon.

Ulcerative proctitis: ulcerative colitis that occurs only in the rectum.

2

Understanding the Diagnosis of Ulcerative Colitis

U lcerative colitis is chronic (long-term: for more than 6 weeks) inflammation of the innermost lining of the colon. This inflammation leads to diarrhea, bleeding, cramping, and urgency. No one understands exactly why ulcerative colitis occurs. There are many theories. As discussed in Chapter 1, it is doubtful that just one thing alone causes ulcerative colitis. Instead, it is likely to be a combination of genes, environment, and something else that triggers the body to start the inflammation process and not shut it off the way it is supposed to. Once the inflammation process has been turned on, it can't be stopped, but it can be controlled. Stopping it would amount to curing it. Many, many scientists are searching for this cure.

In virtually 100% of people with ulcerative colitis, the inflammation starts in the rectum and progresses upward through the colon (Figure 3).

Figure 3. Colon Anatomy

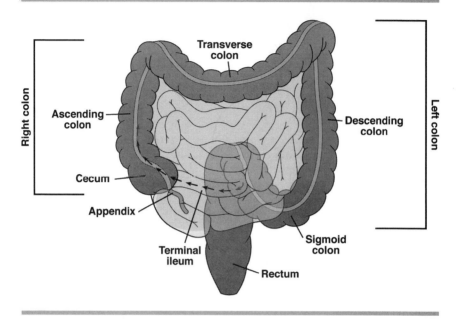

Some people have inflammation only in the rectum; this condition is ulcerative colitis but is called *ulcerative proctitis* to refer to the fact that only the rectum is inflamed. It would be clearer if we called this problem ulcerative "rectitis," but in medicine, we use the Latin term for rectum, which is *procto*.

When the left side of the colon is involved in the inflammation, we call it *left-sided ulcerative colitis,* and when the entire colon is involved, we call it *pancolitis.* At diagnosis, you may have proctitis or left-sided colitis, but over time, the inflammation can progress to involve the entire colon. This progression usually happens within the first two years of diagnosis. Ask the doctor who performed your colonoscopy if biopsies were taken from throughout the entire colon. Sometimes when things look normal we tend not to biopsy those areas. However, under the microscope there may be evidence of subtle inflammation that over time may reveal itself. You may then feel like it "spread," when actually it was there all along but not highly visible. It's important for you to have at least one colonoscopy in which your entire colon is biopsied to find all areas of inflammation.

Symptoms of Ulcerative Colitis

Certain predictable problems occur when there is inflammation of the lining of the colon. Because the parts of the colon that are inflamed no longer absorb water, the most common problem is diarrhea. This occurs because the water that is no longer being absorbed comes out with the stool.

When inflammation continues or becomes worse, it causes the innermost lining of the colon to break down. This damage is called *ulceration*. It's similar to what your skin looks like when you fall down and scrape yourself. You end up with a break in the skin and some bleeding, depending on how hard you fell. These ulcerations bleed, so blood appears in your stool.

Inflammation breaks the normal communication between colon and brain that indicates when you need to have a bowel movement. The rectum has stretch receptors that detect how full the rectum is. Healthy receptors don't detect a stretch until a regular size stool is present and ready to be moved out (evacuated). However, inflammation temporarily damages these stretch signals. It makes them hypersensitive. The result is that, whether there is stool in the rectum or only air, the signal is sent that you need to evacuate *and you need to do it right now.* You're not able to tell whether there is stool or gas present. When you go to the bathroom and pass just gas, or a little mucus or blood, you might have what some doctors call "dry heaves of the rectum." The medical term for this is *tenesmus.* Because of the inflammation, you can't sense the difference between gas, mucus, blood, or stool in the rectum. This leads to false alarms that send you rushing to the bathroom.

Many people with ulcerative colitis notice that they have to go more often in the mornings and that the need decreases throughout the day. I call this the "morning rush hour," and it's natural because we possess reflexes that make the bowels most active within the first few hours after getting up. Understanding that phenomenon may make it easier to plan your day if you know that you will have the majority of your bowel movements in the first 1 to 2 hours after getting out of bed in the morning.

Along with diarrhea, urgency, and bleeding, you can experience cramps. These tend to be worse right around the time you have to move your bowels, because the colon muscles are contracting. The cramps generally get better a few minutes following bowel evacuation. These are bad cramps but normally are not long lasting. Because the pain fibers are on the outside of the bowel and ulcerative colitis is a condition of the inner lining of the bowel, the nerves that sense pain do not become irritated. However, you may experience pain in the anal area from frequent bowel movements and the breakdown of the normal skin there, but this is because of stool frequency and not the inflammation of ulcerative colitis. Other symptoms can include nighttime bowel movements, fever, loss of appetite, and weight loss. Chapter 7 discusses the other parts of the body that can exhibit inflammation associated with ulcerative colitis.

If you have ulcerative colitis only in the rectum (proctitis), constipation is more the issue than diarrhea. This is because when the rectum is inflamed, the rest of the colon tends to slow down to assist the rectum by letting it rest. Passing blood by itself, constipation, and bright red blood along with relatively solid stools are what you will generally experience with proctitis.

When ulcerative colitis is particularly severe, during periods of intense inflammation, you may experience fevers, constant cramping, and abdominal discomfort along with a sense of bloating or abdominal "swelling." Stools are frequent—up to one every hour—and all of them have blood. Nausea and vomiting can also occur when the colon is very severely inflamed. This situation requires hospitalization for close monitoring by health care professionals in all but rare circumstances. Dehydration is dangerous and can occur quickly, and you will need medications and intravenous fluids at the hospital to keep you safe.

Diagnosis of Ulcerative Colitis

Your health care providers will diagnose ulcerative colitis using a combination of a detailed history, physical exam, and testing. A thorough history consists of your answers to many questions to rule out other types of colitis. Tests are usually stool studies, blood work, and then an endoscopic procedure.

For the history, the more detailed information you can provide, the better.

- When did you first notice the symptoms? (In other words, how long has this been going on?)
- Are your symptoms getting worse or just not going away?
- Have you started or stopped any new medications recently, including supplements, vitamins, and other over-the-counter (nonprescription) therapies?
- Have you traveled outside your normal environment?
- Does anyone with whom you have been in recent contact have similar symptoms?
- Have you recently quit smoking?
- Do you have any family members with a diagnosis of ulcerative colitis or Crohn's disease?
- Have you had any rashes, joint aches, or eye problems along with your bowel symptoms?

Blood testing usually consists of a complete blood count to check for anemia and evidence of infection; a chemistry panel to check electrolytes, kidney and liver function, and protein levels; and a sedimentation rate or C-reactive protein, two common tests that indicate active inflammation. There are blood tests that can look for special proteins that have been associated with the presence of either Crohn's disease or ulcerative colitis. These tests, however, should never be done in the absence of other testing because the information they provide is not sufficient to diagnose either disease. But they are helpful in two situations. The first is when you already have been diagnosed with either Crohn's disease or ulcerative colitis, and we are trying to determine which condition you have. The other situation in which these tests are helpful is in determining how aggressive the inflammation of IBD is in young patients.

Stool tests include looking for white blood cells or specific proteins that indicate inflammation and certain bacteria, parasites, or toxins that could explain your current symptoms. Yeast, in particular *Candida,* is normal in the stool and does not indicate a disease.

A diagnosis of ulcerative colitis requires evidence of inflammation in the colon or rectum. This evidence is collected by viewing in addition to taking a sample (biopsy) of the colon lining. During a colonoscopy, the doctor or other trained professional examines the entire colon, so you must prepare the day before with a clear liquid diet and a cleaning solution that you drink. However, some procedures, such as a flexible sigmoidoscopy, can be done in the office without any prep or sedatives. This is a shorter exam and examines the lower third to bottom half of the colon with a thin, flexible tube with a light on the end. It can be done without an oral prep and usually just a couple of enemas. Sometimes, no prep is needed at all when the diarrhea has been bad and there is no solid stool to clean out. These procedures can be performed in the office by an internist, trained nurse practitioner, gastroenterologist, or surgeon.

If you've never had a colonoscopy, know that the prep is actually the roughest part of the procedure. Bowel cleansing is important for a complete and thorough look at the lining of the colon. Table 1 shows the different formulations of preps that are available. Preps that are phosphorus based are not appropriate if you have, or may have, ulcerative colitis. Fleets preps and Osmoprep tablets contain a lot of phosphate, which can actually cause inflammation and confuse the clinical picture.[19] In addition, phosphate-based preps are not safe for those older than age 60 or those with kidney disease. All the preps taste bad, because they have a lot of salt in them that causes water to be excreted from the colon wall to create diarrhea and thus "flush" or cleanse the colon of all stool. These salts are not the same as table salt, so there is no need to worry about your blood pressure going up when you take this. Some doctors have invented their own cocktail of agents that is more palatable, including some that combine Gatorade and powdered laxatives; ask your physician what he or she would choose to use for his or her own colonoscopy

TABLE 1. Colon Cleansing Preparations		
Name	**Form**	**Comment**
GoLytely	1 gallon fluid	
Nu-Lytely	½ gallon fluid	
MoviPrep	½ gallon fluid	Effective agents in general use
CoLyte	1 gallon fluid	
Half-Lytely	½ gallon fluid	
TriLyte	1 gallon fluid	
Osmoprep	32 tablets	Phosphorous based and can lead to kidney problems
Fleets Phosphosoda (may not be available in all areas)	28-ounce bottle	High phosphate content makes it potentially unsafe in UC; has to be taken with adequate amounts of fluid
Magnesium citrate + modified diet	Multiple bottles over 12–16 hours	Following directions exactly is essential for adequate prep

and why. That might help you understand the choice the doctor has made for you.

Intravenous sedatives will keep you comfortable during the colonoscopy. Sedatives are safer than general anesthesia because you are not totally out and in need of a breathing tube, so it's easier for you to recover. The procedure takes about 20 minutes, but can take longer depending on the length of your colon, how "twisted" it is inside your abdominal cavity, and how many biopsies are being taken. Women tend to have "curvier" colons than men because it has to divert around a uterus and ovaries, so women may have a little more discomfort than men during this procedure. Most people tolerate this very well.

Your gastroenterologist or surgeon may choose to use anesthesia, which involves a deeper level of unconsciousness and is given by specially trained providers. It is more costly and potentially more dangerous given its ability to cause a deeper state of sedation but can provide more comfort if you require it. For this, we use propofol, which is the medication made infamous as the drug given to Michael Jackson to "help him sleep." Talk to your health care provider before the procedure to find out what will be used if you are concerned. The goal is to have a safe and comfortable procedure.

The doctor will use a long, flexible tube called a *colonoscope* to examine the colon and the very end of the small intestine, the terminal ileum. The tube has a video camera on the end and channels through which instruments travel to take little pinches—biopsies—of the lining of the colon. These tissue biopsies provide evidence of damage that is caused by chronic inflammation, which is essential for a correct diagnosis. Examination of the tissue under the microscope helps to eliminate other conditions that can sometimes look like ulcerative colitis. To the camera, inflammation and ulceration from any source looks the same, so it is with the microscope that we can best make a diagnosis. When inflammation of the entire colon is severe, the very end of the small intestine, the terminal ileum, can also show signs of inflammation. This is because the valve that separates the colon from the terminal ileum can become weak, and inflammation "backwashes" into the ileum. We actually call this *backwash ileitis.* This suggests a very active, highly inflamed case of ulcerative colitis.

My patient Michael, 31 years old, had been having loose stools for the past 5 years. He didn't think much about his bowel habits, because having to go frequently did not keep him from his work or other daily activities. But then he started to notice bleeding, and at first, he thought it was hemorrhoids because he was not having any pain. Once he started to have some abdominal cramping, he decided to seek medical advice. His doctor sent him for a colonoscopy, after which he was told he had ulcerative colitis. He was started on medications for "colitis" and got better rather quickly, so after a few weeks, he stopped taking the medicine. After all, no one had told him that he had to continue taking the medication even if his symptoms were better. Unfortunately, within a few months' time, the symptoms returned, and he found himself back where he started.

Pat is 75 years old and very overweight, with high cholesterol and high blood pressure. She was recently diagnosed with type 2 diabetes and is facing a hip replacement. Over the past year, she has had episodes of diarrhea and fecal incontinence requiring her to wear adult diapers if she is away from home for any length of time. She had always been a hearty eater and continues to enjoy her favorite foods, not being able to single out which ones might be triggering her distressing condition. Although Pat is a widow and living alone with some money concerns, her sons and their families live nearby.

Pat, like many older people, has a more complex medical condition than younger people usually have. Her body is not as healthy as it once was. This is one of the reasons that it is more difficult to diagnose IBD in older people. Although IBD is most often diagnosed in young people, it is not as rare in the elderly as previously believed. There is a second, smaller peak of IBD diagnoses between ages 60 and 80, and up to 20% of people with ulcerative colitis or Crohn's disease are elderly at the time their symptoms begin. This is a special population with its own set of challenges, beginning with the mistaken idea that IBD doesn't happen to older people.

There are other obstacles to reaching a correct diagnosis of IBD. For Pat, symptoms caused by her diabetes and other conditions get mixed up with possible symptoms of IBD. Her test results may not fall into the categories used for younger patients with IBD, so we can't be clear about what's going on. We don't yet have universal diagnostic criteria that apply equally well to people of all ages.

When I see an older patient like Pat, with new symptoms suggestive of IBD such as bloody diarrhea or abdominal pain, I compile a thorough medical history and consider her other conditions and factors, particularly all the medications she is taking. I eliminate other conditions that can have similar symptoms as IBD, such as:

- ischemic colitis, lack of blood flow to the colon causing damage to the lining
- infection: *Salmonella, Shigella, Campylobacter, Yersinia, C. difficile, E. coli*
- diverticular disease
- microscopic colitis
- radiation colitis
- cancer
- medication use: nonsteroidal anti-inflammatory medications (NSAIDs), gold compounds, ticlopidine, phosphate soda preparations

Atypical symptoms are more common in the elderly with IBD. For instance, an older individual with peripheral vascular disease and high blood pressure may have confusion as a result of diarrhea and dehydration that is the presenting symptom of new IBD. An overlapping *C. difficile* infection may show up as an ileus (slow down of the small intestine so that it does not move) and an elevated white blood cell count rather than diarrhea. Then again, involuntary release of stool (incontinence) is more of an issue with advancing age, because of weakness of the anal sphincter muscles.

I need the patient's help in tracking the symptoms, although he or she may or may not be able to focus on this with me. The presence of other conditions, such as coronary artery disease, high blood pressure, peripheral vascular disease, or diabetes, may mean that the patient is much sicker than my younger patients usually are. That is why elderly patients more often go into the hospital at diagnosis—to be sure they are getting all the care they need.

Pat did indeed have ulcerative colitis, and she began 5-ASA therapy. But her disease did not respond as fast as I would have hoped with 5-ASA therapy, so I was forced to start steroids. This made her diabetes worse, but we managed it with more insulin as we got her colitis under control. Pat was then able to return to 5-ASA therapy, which she has tolerated well. Pat is happy that once again she is able to sit through a bridge game without interference.

Management of Ulcerative Colitis

You may have had months, perhaps years, of symptoms before you were diagnosed with ulcerative colitis. Once diagnosed, however, treatment can begin. One rule of thumb is that the period of time that you have been sick is about how long it may take you to get better. There are very few "quick fixes" in IBD.

Your treatment needs to be individualized to your specific needs. These can include some or all of the following:

- where in the colon the inflammation was found
- how severe and extensive the inflammation is

- whether you have any history of allergies
- your insurance coverage (every insurance company has "preferred" medications that may differ from what your physician wants to prescribe)
- other medical conditions you have
- your personal preferences

Ulcerative colitis therapy is definitely not one-size-fits-all. Two people with the same set of symptoms and severity of ulcerative colitis may be treated in completely different ways depending on their other individual factors.

One thing that is the same for everyone with ulcerative colitis is a twofold goal: first, to get your symptoms under control as quickly and as safely as possible, and second, to keep your symptoms under control. Although there is no cure for ulcerative colitis yet, there are medications that can moderate your symptoms.

The inflammation of colitis can be treated in a variety of ways, and Chapter 6, on medications, has many details. For ulcerative colitis, we treat the location as well as the severity of the disease. Someone with only a few centimeters of disease in the colon can be worse off than someone with mild symptoms involving the entire colon. If there is inflammation that requires several courses of steroids, this is the "tipping point" that signals the need for more aggressive therapy. Make sure you have discussed with your health care provider an "exit strategy" to get you off the steroids once you have started. Please know that it is possible to heal the colon lining so that it looks normal, and even under the microscope, it is not as inflamed.

Flares

Many patients have told me, "I have been feeling well for such a long time that I don't need my medicine any more." I wish that were true. If you stop using your medication, the symptoms will return eventually. We call these "flares," which refers to the return of the inflammation.

It's true that some people can go into remission and stay off their medicines, some for as long as a few years. Unfortunately, this is a slim minority of people with ulcerative colitis and, even then, ulcerative colitis does flare up again. A recent Internet survey of people with ulcerative colitis revealed that, on average, they have six to eight flares per year.[20] However, only a fraction of those flares are reported to their doctor. Most people treat the flares themselves and don't necessarily recognize the pattern of repeated flares.

Not all flares are caused by stopping or reducing your ulcerative colitis medications. There are other culprits. It's clear that certain antibiotics can cause a flare, including the group of antibiotics in the penicillin family (amoxicillin, ampicillin). If you are prescribed one of these antibiotics, discuss with the doctor why it may be necessary. Most of the time, a penicillin alternative can work just as well with no risk of a flare.

Traveling can disrupt your normal routine and cause a flare, as can acute illnesses like the flu or a sinus infection. Most patients report a seasonal variation to their symptoms, particularly spring (April) and fall (October).[21] We are not entirely sure why this occurs, but it is a well-documented phenomenon. Smoking cessation makes ulcerative colitis worse, a connection that baffles the medical community.[22] People with ulcerative colitis are more likely to be ex-smokers or nonsmokers. And then there is stress, an important factor that I discuss further in Chapter 11.[23] Finally, use of the acne medication Accutane has rarely been associated with both the development of ulcerative colitis and flares of disease.[24] This risk is very small and is outweighed by the potential benefit of treating severe acne. If your dermatologist has recommended Accutane for your acne, discuss this in advance with your IBD physician and make sure it is the right choice for you. For most people, it's a good choice, but you will need to monitor your ulcerative colitis symptoms. If they worsen, let your physician know what's happening.

Please look at your ulcerative colitis as a chronic condition, similar to diabetes or hypertension. You can control it with the medicines you take and with healthy lifestyle choices. The more you know, the better you will be at self-managing the ulcerative colitis.

3

Understanding the Diagnosis of Crohn's Disease

C rohn's disease is chronic inflammation of any part of the GI tract and involves all the layers of the bowel wall (called *transmural*). These characteristics are the defining difference between Crohn's disease and ulcerative colitis. Ulcerative colitis involves only the inner layer of the large intestine and disease is confined to that area.

The GI tract (Figure 4) starts in the mouth and consists of the esophagus; stomach; small intestine (duodenum, jejunum, and ileum); colon (large intestine or bowel); rectum; and anus. The terminal ileum is the last few inches of the ileum.

About a third of people with Crohn's disease have inflammation of just their small intestine. Another third have inflammation of their small intestine and colon, and the last third have inflammation of only

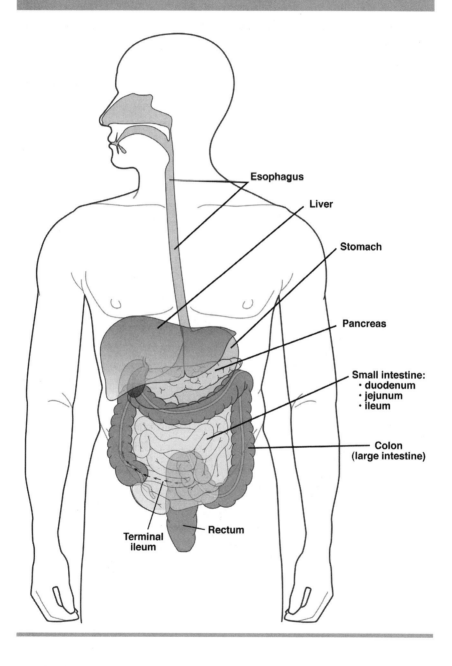

FIGURE 4. Gastrointestinal Tract

Esophagus

Liver

Stomach

Pancreas

Small intestine:
· duodenum
· jejunum
· ileum

Colon
(large intestine)

Terminal
ileum

Rectum

their colon. Regardless of the location, the inflammation of Crohn's disease penetrates all layers of the bowel walls (Figure 5).

When I met Melissa, she was 28 years old, but she'd had "stomach problems" since childhood. Her first surprise was to learn that she was anemic, although everyone assumed it was due to her periods. When she started having really bad abdominal pain, she thought that she had better check things out. A computed tomography (CT) scan showed thickening of her small intestine, and a colonoscopy showed inflammation in her right colon and terminal ileum. Melissa

FIGURE 5. Intestine and Colon Walls Cross-Sections

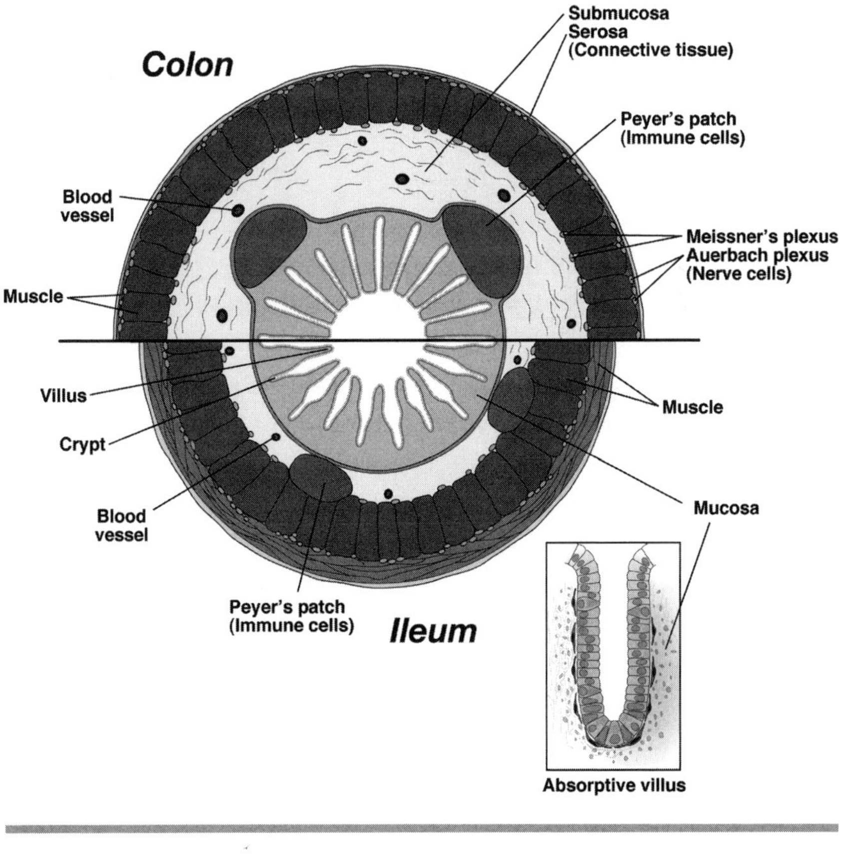

Colon

Submucosa
Serosa
(Connective tissue)

Peyer's patch
(Immune cells)

Blood vessel

Meissner's plexus
Auerbach plexus
(Nerve cells)

Muscle

Villus

Muscle

Crypt

Blood vessel

Mucosa

Peyer's patch
(Immune cells)

Ileum

Absorptive villus

was diagnosed with Crohn's disease. This was devastating news, as the only exposure she had to Crohn's disease was the mother of one of her close friends, who had died of complications during a hospitalization. Obviously upset and scared, Melissa had a lot to learn about her disease and the hopeful outlook that she had for a full, prolonged life.

Types of Crohn's Disease

There are three "types" of Crohn's disease: inflammatory, fistulizing, and fibrostenosing. Almost all people with IBD, whether it is Crohn's disease or ulcerative colitis, begin by having only inflammation of some portion of the gastrointestinal tract. Over time, however, about 30% of these individuals experience inflammation that burrows through all of the layers of the bowel wall and causes a fistula, or abnormal connection, to another part of the body.[25] A fistula can be internal, meaning that it's entirely on the inside of the body, such as a connection from one piece of bowel to another piece of bowel. This may not cause any symptoms, so it might only be noticed in an X-ray. In the third type of Crohn's, when inflammation continues to "smolder" over time, scar tissue builds up and creates a thickening of the affected part of the bowel. This thickening causes narrowing of the bowel (stenosis) by fibrous scar tissue. This is the fibrostenosing type of Crohn's disease. This happens in only about 10% of people with Crohn's. Most people with Crohn's disease have inflammation without the other issues. However, some start out with inflammation and progress to another type of Crohn's disease.

Health care professionals label the types of Crohn's disease by location and character. For instance, someone with disease that is limited to inflammation in the large bowel would have *Crohn's colitis.* Someone with inflammation in the small intestine and no evidence of narrowing or fistula would be said to have *inflammatory Crohn's ileitis.* Someone with a fistula between the small intestine and colon with inflammation in both locations would have *fistulizing ileocolitis.*

Symptoms of Crohn's Disease

With Crohn's disease, your symptoms will vary widely depending on where the inflammation is, how severe the inflammation is, and even your own perception of the symptoms themselves. Because the most common location is at the end of the small intestine, the most common symptoms at first are abdominal pain, diarrhea that can occur both during the day and at night, fatigue, nausea, and sometimes vomiting, along with weight loss.

Sharon, a 17-year-old, was having pain after meals, which she described as crampy or sharp and usually at the right lower side of her abdomen. One night it got so bad that her parents brought her to the emergency department of their hospital. Due to the location of the pain, the doctors suspected that she had appendicitis and ordered a CT scan of her abdomen. Sharon's appendix looked normal but the last few inches of the small intestine (terminal ileum) were swollen and ulcerated, suggesting that she might have Crohn's disease instead.

If you experience bleeding, this is because the colon walls are affected by the inflammation and have been damaged enough that they bleed. This is similar to bleeding that might occur from your skin if you fell and scraped your knee. However, many patients with Crohn's disease do not experience any bleeding.

As symptoms continue, you could have more weight loss, along with fevers and joint pains. Pediatricians might diagnose failure to grow; this is often the first sign of Crohn's disease in children (see Chapter 12). When Crohn's disease occurs in the esophagus, which is relatively uncommon, the symptoms may include difficulty swallowing or pain with swallowing. Crohn's disease in the jejunum usually results in pain in the middle of the abdomen, with a lot of bloating, gas, and watery diarrhea. As you can see, Crohn's disease results in a wide variety of symptoms.

Tad's story is a good example. Tad, a 20-year-old college student, was always "small for his age." As he was more of a computer nerd than athlete, this didn't bother him. What did bother him were "big" meals. After eating, he would have a lot of bloating, loose runny stools, and nausea. When he started college and watched his friends eat, he realized that he wasn't overeating after all. Even normal portions of food affected him, and once he realized this, he made a visit to the college clinic. It turned out that Tad had Crohn's disease of the jejunum, and that his being small was really growth failure caused by the disease harming his intestine. His inability to eat large meals came from the narrowed, scarred intestine that would cause blockages when he ate.

Diagnosis of Crohn's Disease

Because the symptoms for Crohn's disease are not specific and could result from many different conditions, medical evaluation is absolutely necessary to make the correct diagnosis. The diagnosis starts with a complete history and physical exam. The more detailed and complete a list of your history and symptoms that you can share with your health care provider, the better.

- When did you first notice the symptoms? (In other words, how long has this been going on?)
- Are your symptoms getting worse, or just not going away?
- Have you started or stopped any new medications recently, including supplements, vitamins, and other over-the-counter (nonprescription) therapies?
- Have you traveled outside your normal environment?
- Does anyone with whom you have been in recent contact have similar symptoms?
- What surgeries have you had?
- Are you a smoker?
- Do you have any family members with a diagnosis of ulcerative colitis or Crohn's disease?
- Have you had any rashes, joint aches, or eye problems along with your bowel symptoms?

First, you'll need a complete physical. This evaluates all body parts, even those seemingly not directly involved with your current symptoms, because they may provide clues about what is causing your problems. A rectal exam is part of the physical, because many patients with Crohn's disease have "skin tags" or hemorrhoids around the anal canal that can suggest inflammation. Narrowing or cracks in the anal canal can also be clues for Crohn's disease. Sometimes, the rectal exam is performed during a colonoscopy, so that it can be done more thoroughly while you're sedated.

The location of your symptoms will steer what tests the doctor decides to do. Most agree, however, that everyone starts with basic blood tests that include a blood count; iron studies to rule out deficiency; chemistry panel to assess electrolytes, kidney and liver function, and protein levels; thyroid hormone levels; and sedimentation rate or C-reactive protein, two common tests that indicate active inflammation.

Some tests look for special proteins (commonly called *markers*) that have been associated with the presence of either Crohn's disease or ulcerative colitis. These tests, however, should never be done in the absence of other testing because they do not provide enough information to diagnose Crohn's disease or ulcerative colitis. But they are helpful in two situations. The first is when someone already has been diagnosed with either condition, and we are trying to determine which condition they have. The other situation where these tests are helpful is in determining how aggressive the inflammation of Crohn's disease or colitis is in young patients.[26] The markers are proteins that your body produces as a reaction to certain common bacteria and carbohydrates that normally are found in our bodies. It is unclear why someone would react to specific bacteria or carbohydrates and not others, and the overall significance of these markers in the inflammatory process is unknown. At this time, the use of these markers is still in the research phase, and so they are not applicable to standard care.

We also do stool studies to look for blood, bacteria, parasites, and the toxin produced by the bacterium *Clostridium difficile*. Stool may also be checked for fat content, which suggests it's not being properly absorbed by the small intestine, or white blood cells, which signal inflammation. Finally, the stool sample will be used to measure protein content. Certain proteins appear in the stool when inflammation is active. Calprotectin and lactoferrin are proteins that are such sensitive markers of inflammation that, if they are absent in stool, we can be certain that no inflammation is occurring.[27, 28]

Finally, we want to look at your digestive tract. Our basic imaging tools are X-rays, including plain films, usually to rule out obstruction; barium studies; computerized axial tomography (CT or CAT) scans; and magnetic resonance imaging (MRI). Barium is a contrast agent that helps us visualize the structures in the gut. Plain barium studies ("upper GI" and "small bowel follow through") are somewhat old-fashioned and outdated now but still can serve a purpose in certain situations, such as outlining a long narrowing of the intestine (stricture). There are several forms of CAT scans. There is a plain CT where no contrast or dye is given, which is done to rule out swelling (abscess) or abnormal opening or tear (perforation). It is used widely in emergency departments and for patients with kidney diseases who should not be exposed to the contrast. For most CAT scans, you need to drink barium, although it is a thinner formula than needed in the past. CT enterography (CTE) is relatively new and involves drinking a large volume of even thinner barium, which helps us to really focus on the details of the wall of the small intestine. CTE is not uniformly available as of yet but gaining in popularity as the test of choice when Crohn's disease is being considered or evaluated.[29]

Another kind of specialized X-ray exam is called an *enteroclysis*. This is a very unpleasant test and not ordered frequently, but it can definitely be helpful in certain situations. In particular, it helps us find the source of problems for those patients who continue to have symptoms of obstruction like nausea, vomiting, and pain with the inability to pass stool or gas, where standard X-rays have not revealed the source. This technique can be done by either CT or MRI and involves drinking contrast, after which a thin tube is passed through the nose or mouth down into the stomach to pump air into the entire small intestine. With the small intestine inflated, we can find any blocked areas.

Doctors use several different imaging techniques in diagnosing Crohn's disease. When you have X-rays, CT scans, or MRI of your abdomen, what are the doctors looking for? They are looking for several problems:

- evidence that you have inflammation or swelling of the wall of the intestine
- craters in the intestine wall, which can signal the presence of ulcers
- tracks of contrast dye outside the bowel, which may indicate an abnormal connection between two body parts (fistula)
- a narrowing of the intestine, which suggests an obstruction (stenosis)
- an area above a narrowing that is dilated from chronic stretching of bowel due to stool having to sit before it can move through the narrow area

X-rays and CT scans use radiation for imaging, and some work best using a contrast dye to maximize the details seen. But the more of these you have, the higher your exposure to radiation. Health care providers are aware of the importance of limiting radiation exposure. MRI uses no radiation and is good for seeing fat and muscle and is also helpful in finding fistulas and abscesses. MRI is a very good option for someone who may need repeated exams over a relatively short amount of time. The downside is that in many cases, contrast dye is still needed, and your liver will need to clear it from your body. Also, because of the configuration of the MRI machine, if you are prone to claustrophobia, you may find these tests difficult.

X-rays and scans provide images that we can read, but to actually see the inside of your digestive tract, we use endoscopy. Endoscopy is a very important way for your doctor to obtain a first-hand look at the lining of your intestine and get tissue biopsies. Colonoscopy with examination of the terminal ileum is essential in Crohn's diagnosis, and an upper endoscopy of the stomach and first part of the small intestine is done frequently when someone has symptoms that suggest inflammation or irritation in the stomach, like nausea, heartburn, or dyspepsia (the feeling of an upset stomach).

Video capsule endoscopy (the "pill camera") is used to assess the status of existing Crohn's disease. More and more insurance companies are now paying for it to be used in diagnosing suspected Crohn's. After your doctor confirms that you have no narrowings that can trap it, you swallow a capsule that is the size of a large vitamin. You wear a belt that captures images taken by the camera as it moves through the intestine. These images are studied like a movie. The camera can be very sensitive, and even small ulcers and breaks in the intestine lining can be seen.

Why would we do one kind of test over the other? Here's what I tell my patients. A regular CT scan lets you look at the whole body as if you were flying over the Grand Canyon in a commercial jet. You get an idea of how big it is but not a lot of detail. If you have a CT scan with a barium contrast dye, it's like seeing the Grand Canyon from a helicopter—in much more detail and closer up. An endoscopy or video capsule study is like being on the Colorado River in a raft where you are actually inside the Canyon.

Management of Crohn's Disease

The nature of Crohn's disease is that it waxes and wanes. This means that there are periods of active disease (a waxing or buildup) interspersed with periods of disease remission (the waning part). Our goal is to maximize the amount of time you spend in remission and minimize the number and duration of flares. Keep in mind that if you have been sick for some time before diagnosis and treatment, it may take nearly the same amount of time for you to reach a period of remission. There are very few "quick fixes" in IBD.

How often you get flares and how long they last depends on several factors. First, the location of your inflammation is going to drive what symptoms you get. (See "Symptoms," page 35.) Although flares can seem to come on randomly, there are several known triggers. Stopping your medications will lead to flares. If your medications are keeping your disease in remission, then you have to stay on them. Try to see Crohn's disease as it is: an incurable but treatable chronic disease, like diabetes. If you have diabetes that is controlled by insulin, you keep taking insulin. If your blood glucose test is in the normal range, that doesn't mean you can stop taking insulin—it means that the treatment is working.

Certain antibiotics can cause a flare, including the group of antibiotics in the penicillin family. Traveling can cause disruption to your normal routine and cause a flare, as can contracting an illness such as the flu or a sinus infection. Smoking makes Crohn's disease worse, so it's very important to quit (or never start smoking). Then, there is stress. The role of stress in flares is controversial, and I discuss this further in Chapter 11. Finally, use of the acne medication Accutane has rarely been associated with both the development of Crohn's disease and flares.[24] This risk is very small and is outweighed by the potential benefit of treating severe acne. If your dermatologist has recommended Accutane for your acne, discuss this in advance with your IBD physician and make sure it is the right choice for you. For most people, it's a good choice, but you will need to monitor your Crohn's disease symptoms. If they worsen, let your physician know what's happening.

Crohn's disease does not "spread," although it's often described that way if someone is trying to give a simple explanation. In reality, Crohn's disease involves whatever part of the body it is going to affect within the first year of the diagnosis. If after a year, other parts of the GI tract suddenly develop symptoms, be certain that the disease was already present there, but that area may not have been evaluated because there were no symptoms. It simply was just missed at diagnosis. After surgery, we find that Crohn's disease recurs exactly where it was before, so in that sense it has not "spread" either (see Chapter 9). We have yet to understand how Crohn's recurs after a piece of affected bowel is removed.

You know your body better than anyone else. If you are experiencing symptoms that involve the GI tract but they feel different than your usual flare, speak up. Having Crohn's disease does not make you immune to getting other illnesses, like food poisoning, stomach flu, or a side effect from a medication. For example, let's say that you have Crohn's disease in your colon and for you a normal flare is diarrhea and bleeding. But one day you develop nausea and vomiting. Nausea and vomiting is a common combination of symptoms but it should not automatically be assumed to be a symptom of your Crohn's disease. This is a common mistake. I have even missed the diagnosis of pregnancy in a young woman who had persistent nausea because I was so focused on her Crohn's disease!

4

The Other Types of IBD

Indeterminate Colitis

About 10% of people with inflammatory bowel disease in the colon have what we call *indeterminate colitis*.[30] This means that they have features of both Crohn's disease and ulcerative colitis. But it does not mean that they have both diseases. If you have been diagnosed with indeterminate colitis, you have inflammation of the colon that is difficult to distinguish between the two diagnoses. Sometimes even experts have a hard time determining what is Crohn's disease and what is ulcerative colitis.

Remember, the term *colitis* simply means inflammation of the colon. Most people use colitis to refer to ulcerative colitis, but Crohn's disease of the colon is still colitis: it is Crohn's colitis. The management is the same regardless of which name you want to give it—because it is inflammation of the colon. Sometimes, over the span of years, the colitis "declares" itself as either ulcerative colitis or Crohn's disease because the nature of it or character of the symptoms changes somehow. However, studies show that people with indeterminate colitis continue to have features of both diseases and never really change, even after 7 to 10 years of having the disease.

Jennifer is a 24-year-old who began to notice a change in her bowel habits a few years ago. She saw blood in her stools and had some weight loss, along with cramping and diarrhea. A colonoscopy revealed inflammation throughout her entire colon, but her rectum actually looked pretty normal. Some of the ulcers noted were very deep, as if they were penetrating into the deeper layers of the colon wall. A CT scan did not show any thickening of her small intestine. She did have some hemorrhoids also, which was contributing to her bleeding. Because it was hard to determine whether Jennifer had ulcerative colitis or Crohn's disease limited to the colon, she was diagnosed with indeterminate colitis. The fact that it was throughout the colon and no areas appeared normal suggested ulcerative colitis, but the deeper ulcers and relative normal appearance of the rectum suggested Crohn's disease.

Because ulcerative colitis is confined to the colon, some say that any inflammation found in the small intestine (ileum) must be a sign that it is Crohn's disease. However, inflammation in the colon can be so bad that it causes the valve that seals off the small intestine from the colon to become inflamed also, and some of the inflammation can "backwash" into the ileum. This inflammation is not the same as the inflammation of Crohn's disease. Sometimes, a pathologist (specialist in the diseases of cells) is needed to determine which disease is present.

Some health care providers use specific protein markers in the blood to try to distinguish between the two conditions. People with colitis (either ulcerative colitis or Crohn's colitis) are more likely to have the protein p-ANCA in their blood than the rest of the population. ASCA, another marker, is more common in people with Crohn's disease, regardless of where their disease is located. And there are even more specific proteins used to separate ulcerative colitis from Crohn's disease. But none of them are useful for diagnosis without other testing like endoscopy with biopsy.

Microscopic or Lymphocytic Colitis

Microscopic colitis is considered to be an inflammatory bowel disease because it involves inflammation of the colon lining. This condition, however, does not cause the ulceration seen in ulcerative colitis. It is called *microscopic colitis* because it is only seen under the microscope.[31] When a patient has a colonoscopy, the lining appears totally normal. It is only when biopsy tissue samples are examined under the microscope that abnormal inflammation is seen. It is called *lymphocytic colitis* also, because certain white blood cells called *lymphocytes* cause the inflammation.

Microscopic colitis mainly affects women. It can be a result of an allergic-type reaction to a medicine, or it can happen for unclear reasons. Certain medications, such as an anti-inflammatory like ibuprofen, acid-reducing medications like proton pump inhibitors, and high blood pressure medicines, are most likely to cause this condition.

At age 60, Mary Jane's life has been turned upside down by six months of bad diarrhea. She is going as much as 12 times a day and waking up at night to use the toilet as well. She has not seen any blood and has not lost any weight, although she cannot understand why not, considering all the diarrhea. She has seen her primary doctor, who suggested that she increase her fiber intake to bulk up her stools, which did not help at all. She had a colonoscopy performed by a local surgeon, who found no evidence for active inflammation and no tumors or polyps. She was told it was "all in her head" and to take Imodium as needed when she was planning to go out. Unsatisfied, Mary Jane came to see me for another colonoscopy. An examination of her rectum and sigmoid colon was normal; however, when the biopsies from these areas were examined under the microscope, they showed that Mary Jane had chronic inflammation typical of microscopic colitis. After 10 days on the appropriate anti-inflammatory medication for this condition, she was back to having solid stools, and her life once again returned to normal.

Microscopic colitis causes a watery diarrhea, sometimes up to 15 to 20 stools per day. There is no blood because there is no ulceration of the intestine lining. Usually there is no weight loss either, and as it was for Mary Jane, the correct diagnosis can take a while. Some individuals respond to treatment with medications that relieve diarrhea but others need the medicines used to treat ulcerative colitis to get the inflammation under control. This type of colitis can actually disappear completely in some people. It is very helpful, of course, if you can identify which medication was responsible.

Collagenous Colitis

One of the important parts of the bowel wall, which gives it structure and strength, is the layer of collagen (Figure 5, page 33). For some reason, in some people this layer overgrows and becomes thicker. We believe that an inflammatory process may make this happen. When the collagen layer becomes too thick, it prevents water from re-entering the colon wall, which is the main function of the colon. Unabsorbed water leads to watery diarrhea. There is no blood in the stool because there is no ulceration. This diagnosis also can only be made by examining intestinal wall biopsy tissue samples under the microscope for a thickened collagen layer. The lining appears normal in all other ways.

Women are also more likely to have this condition and, as with microscopic colitis, will have watery but not bloody diarrhea. Pepto-Bismol shrinks the collagen layer back to normal in a certain percentage of patients, and others respond to common antidiarrheal medicines.[32] For those who do not respond, the anti-inflammatory medications used to treat ulcerative colitis are also used for this condition.

5

Self-Management: It's Your IBD

How inflammatory bowel disease affects you is an individual matter. The theme in this book is that one size does not fit all, so there is no one recipe for how you take care of your IBD. You could think of IBD management as an ongoing discussion between you and your health care professionals. They make treatment recommendations, and you provide feedback on what worked and what didn't. Then together you pinpoint your challenges and goals and discuss what to do next.

This means that your active involvement is necessary. Consider that your team needs to learn from you how you want to manage IBD on your terms. You need to learn what your health care professionals recommend as appropriate management for you. As for me, I feel strongly that I am here to help my patients but not to enable them to use IBD as an excuse to give up or drop out of life.

It is a team effort, and there is no single correct way to go about managing your IBD. But we need to start somewhere. There are some important milestones, such as diagnosis or worsening of symptoms, that require active medical management. I want to share with you the kinds of management decisions I discuss with my patients at each important milestone in their disease.

In my first meetings with a patient, I usually have three types of plans in mind: one immediate, one short term, and one long term. What you and I generally want to do right away is deal with the one or two major symptoms that you are experiencing—often it's the pain and diarrhea. If you were just diagnosed, then the emphasis is different than if you have had IBD for some time and are experiencing a flare.

The Immediate Plan

Let's start with the scenario that you have just been diagnosed and are in the office for a discussion about your test results. The first thing to determine is: Do you need to be in the hospital for treatment, or are you stable enough to go home with a treatment plan and take care of yourself? To make this decision, we would discuss how much inflammation the tests revealed and the location. This would give us an idea of how much damage was occurring and help you understand why you were having particular, specific symptoms.

Whether you have a hospital stay or go home, the next part of the immediate plan centers on choices for medication. There are medications that suppress the inflammation and help treat the symptoms and some medications that just do one or the other. If you are hospitalized, treatment includes intravenous medications like steroids, antibiotics, and fluids. We know someone is stable enough to go home when they are able to take in adequate fluids and calories to sustain themselves, and the bleeding and diarrhea are perhaps not gone but are a fraction of what they were.

The main categories of medications used are listed below:

Medication	Action	Used For
Steroids	Potent anti-inflammatory	IBD
Antibiotics	Anti-infection	Crohn's disease
Aminosalicylates	Anti-inflammatory	Ulcerative colitis and some Crohn's disease
Immunomodulators	Anti-inflammatory .	IBD
Biologics	Anti-inflammatory	IBD

Whenever you begin a new medication, it's important to follow up with your health care provider within two weeks to discuss the results. That's the only way to know whether the treatment plan is working and you are tolerating the medication that was prescribed. There are several reasons why the plan may not be working.

- The medication may not be strong enough for the level of disease activity you have. We usually want to start with a medication that has limited side effects and hope that it will be enough to manage the inflammation.
- Your disease may be more active than we thought. Patients sometimes minimize their symptoms so as to not appear like a "wimp," in which case the chosen therapy may not be effective.
- You may be having side effects that keep you from taking the amount of medication that you need.
- Not enough time has passed for you to get the full benefits of the medication.
- Some other confounding factor that is not allowing for results, such as an ongoing or overlapping infection.

If you are allergic to the medication or are dealing with a bad side effect, or it is simply too expensive to be on the medication, we want to discuss this early, before it appears to me that you are getting benefit from the medication and doing fine. This is time for complete honesty with your health care provider about how you are doing.

For someone who is diagnosed with Crohn's disease and a fistula, the immediate plan may include surgery. Kevin was feeling pretty poorly when he arrived at his hospital's emergency room with a three-day history of worsening abdominal pain, fevers, nausea, and vomiting. He had been at a friend's cookout a few days earlier and assumed that he had food poisoning. A CT scan revealed a large abscess in his lower right side and a lot of inflamed bowel. He went to the operating room, where the surgeon drained the abscess, removed the piece of inflamed bowel, and sewed him back together. Within a few days, Kevin saw that there was stool draining from a tiny hole on the outside of his skin where his surgical scar was. He had developed a fistula (opening) from a portion of the inflamed bowel that was still inside him to the outside world. When Kevin came to me for a second opinion about managing his Crohn's disease, he required a second surgery.

Many times, this immediate care is in conjunction with a surgeon if the fistula is in the perianal or vaginal area or draining directly from the abdominal wall. After a surgical procedure, you will follow up by having exams to assess how well the wound is closing and to be educated on what you need to do to keep it closed.

The Short-Term Plan

The two weeks between a new prescription or treatment approach and the return visit mark the transition from the immediate plan to the short-term plan. The short-term plan may be as simple as continuing with the current medication regimen or increasing the dose if you are tolerating it but not having the kind of response we expect. We may need to add another medication, for the short term, to achieve the desired response. We may need to taper the dose of a short-term medication (for example, steroids) if you had received the intended effect or if side effects are keeping you from taking as much as you really need (for example, with sulfasalazine).

If the medications are working as intended, then the short-term plan may involve testing. For example, I would want to check your nutritional and bone health with tests that are generally not done specifically for an IBD diagnosis, like vitamin levels and a bone density scan. This kind of information might identify ways to improve your long-term health with different food choices or supplements and indicate whether visiting a dietitian would be helpful.

Kathy, age 35, has Crohn's disease, smokes cigarettes, and is constantly eating out because she travels for work quite a bit. She came in complaining of cramping and bloating, and told me she sometimes can see undigested food in her stools. A recent colonoscopy did not show any active disease, and she has been diligent about taking her medications. However, Kathy eats whatever is convenient while on the road and pays the price. She met with a dietitian to help her make better food choices when traveling. The next time I saw her, she told me that her cramping and bloating had improved because she was avoiding certain foods, like tacos with refried beans and caffeine after 4:00 p.m.

Also, it's a good time to get you up to date on vaccinations—especially if you are taking medications that suppress your immune system. Before starting an immunosuppressant or immunomodulator, double-check about whether you are up to date on your tetanus vaccine and, if appropriate, your hepatitis vaccine status. Getting the flu vaccine annually is highly recommended, too.

Information Overload

There is so much to know about living with IBD. And we learn something new every month about treating Crohn's disease and ulcerative colitis. But if you are presented with too much information at once, it can feel overwhelming, and there is only so much you can take in and use right away. Because our knowledge is growing so rapidly, what you were taught years ago about IBD might no longer be exactly correct! My advice is to learn what you need to know right now, and stay curious—learn at your own speed and to suit your own needs.

There are high-quality, reliable sources of information to turn to when you are ready to learn something new. Updated, credible information is found at the Crohn's & Colitis Foundation of America (CCFA, www.ccfa.org), the National Institutes of Health (www.nih.gov), and the Foundation for Clinical Research in Inflammatory Bowel Disease (www.myibd.org). Other sources include WebMD and UpToDate (www.uptodate.com/patients/index.html) and sites created by various universities, gastroenterology practices, and pharmaceutical companies. All sources vary in their biases and ability to be timely, so I encourage you to discuss the information, particularly concerning medications, with your health care provider. This is part of the ongoing conversation of living with IBD.

Your Self-Awareness Tool

Have you considered keeping a diary of your symptoms, linked to when and what you eat, your activities, and if you are a woman, your menstrual cycle? This information will give you and your health care provider valuable insight on your unique patterns and habits that will help you self-manage your IBD. I also suggest that you list your test results and your medications, with dates and doses (Figure 6). This will prevent you from undergoing tests that you may have recently had or retaking medications that did not work just because you don't remember the name of them. And of course, this is really valuable information when you see a new health care provider.

Another component of the short-term plan is to discuss realistic timelines for improvement and for you to see a response from your ther-

FIGURE 6. Sample Symptom Diary			
Date	**Symptom**	**Activity before Symptom**	**Action Taken**
June 21	Diarrhea	Ate at local diner	Took Imodium
July 3	Abdominal pain	Ate at picnic	Lay down

apy. The medications chapter (Chapter 6) describes in detail most of the therapies currently in use for Crohn's disease and ulcerative colitis. Involving loved ones at this time can be important so that early on in the disease process they can learn as well. I encourage my patients to bring along a spouse, friend, or relative to the first few appointments.

The short-term plan may include surgery. This was the case with Mark, a 48-year-old auto repair shop manager who had been diagnosed with ulcerative colitis about three months earlier. At the time, he was having 10 to 12 bloody bowel movements per day and rapidly began to lose weight. Mark was hospitalized once, at his diagnosis, and treated with intravenous steroids. He was discharged from the hospital on oral steroids, but he never really got better. Mark continued to have multiple bloody stools per day and more weight loss. By the time he came to see me, he had lost 20% of his original body weight and could hardly walk on his own power. He was anemic, malnourished, and miserable. There was little that steroids were going to do to save this badly inflamed colon, and we recommended surgery to remove it.

Surgery can be a very scary proposition, but the course of the disease may have been more rapid than you realized. These are the patients who will do poorly (and may even die) if they delay surgery. Good management involves discussing openly any fears of surgery and making clear that medications do have their limitations.

As you start to see improvement and begin to feel better, the short-term plan expands to include lifestyle and quality of life issues. It's time for us to discuss some appropriate changes in how you eat or your work or school schedule, and also issues that may be on your mind about intimacy, family planning, and all the "what ifs." If your health care provider understands where you are in your life, he or she can help with decisions regarding the appropriateness of medications and timing of follow-up appointments.

It's also time to visit your primary care physician and catch him or her up on your IBD diagnosis and treatment plan. Not every health issue will be IBD related, and it's typical for your gastroenterology care to be focused on your IBD. It generally won't address other issues like colds, flu, backaches, or sprained ankles. Your gastroenterologist may be able to handle every health-related problem, but a specialist is just that—specially trained in a particular area of medicine. Your primary care doctor is trained in more general kinds of care. You need both kinds of medical care.

The Long-Term Plan

Once we have decided on the type of treatment and goals for your IBD therapy, the long-term plan kicks in. This is all about maintaining your remission from inflammation and keeping you in the best general health. So we will work to identify factors that can cause a disease flare, develop a plan for health care maintenance, and try to maximize your health-related quality of life. Quality of life issues involve your goals, like raising a family, finishing school, working, and having relationships. Over time, quality of life issues change and so do personal dynamics, and it is important to realize the ways in which your quality of life affects your health.

It is the information in the rest of this book that will help you really understand what *self-management* of your disease means. Education will enable you to have meaningful discussions with your health care providers about what you are experiencing and help you identify and state your preferences in terms of immediate, short-term, and long-term care.

Your Health Care Team

Because you are living with a chronic disease, you will do best if you have a team of medical professionals to consult with, whether you need a general physical or quick help with a sudden urgent issue. I think you need a primary care doctor to work with you on your general health issues and a gastroenterologist who specializes in IBD. Either doctor may entrust your regular care to a nurse practitioner (NP) or physician assistant (PA), although the NPs and PAs in your gastroenterologist's office will be specially trained in GI issues.

I urge you to find medical professionals with whom you can have a helpful, informative conversation. Find health care professionals who are both good listeners and good teachers. This is your body and you have IBD, so to properly take care of yourself, there's a good chance that you will eventually need to be able to discuss private and often embarrassing things—stool coming from abnormal places or uncomfortable intercourse. If you feel more comfortable talking to either a woman or a man, then actively seek one out to manage your care. However, only about 15% of all practicing gastroenterologists are women.

Your Primary Care Physician

I want you to take good care of your whole body, not just focus only on your IBD (although, understandably, it demands your full attention from time to time). Please don't overlook the rest of your body just because your Crohn's disease or ulcerative colitis is being treated. Women with IBD can get cancer, and men with IBD can have heart attacks or strokes, and vice versa.

You need a general practice health care provider, one who can look beyond your IBD at other health issues. Find a primary care provider who will take a holistic approach to your general health. Having someone help you watch your health both in general and for specific issues becomes even more important as you get older. Most young people, even those with IBD, are relatively healthy.

Your "go-to" doctor may be a general practitioner or an internist. Both are medical doctors with training in all fields of medicine. This person may have been the one who made the first steps toward getting you a diagnosis of IBD and may be very helpful in your ongoing care. In some areas of the country, internists do the bulk of the care of those with IBD and may refer you to a GI specialist only when your condition is very complicated or specialized tests are needed. A good relationship with your primary care physician is as important as with others who may specialize in treating Crohn's disease or ulcerative colitis.

You are a product of your genes; if there is a family history of heart disease, you inherited that risk also. Atherosclerosis from elevated cholesterol still kills more people in the United States than any other cause, and you're not immune just because you have another medical condition. If your IBD treatment includes steroids, which can lead to diabetes and hypertension, your cholesterol levels, blood pressure, and blood glucose should all be checked frequently and at age-appropriate times (Table 2). The same goes for the more common cancers for which Americans are screened. Women should have mammograms starting at age 40, and men should have PSA levels tested starting at age 50.

Many people with IBD mistakenly believe that they should not receive any vaccines. This is not true. The vaccines that people with IBD must avoid are those that are made up of live viruses, like polio, yellow fever, chicken pox, and rotavirus. If any of these are needed, they should be given prior to initiation of any steroids, immunosuppressants, or biologics. Once you are on these medications, the immune system is not able to properly respond to the vaccine, so it won't offer you any protection from those diseases. Vaccines against pneumonia, influenza (the "flu"), tetanus, and hepatitis are still effective and safe and are very important to protect your health. Contracting one of these infections could lead to an inflammatory bout and or could prolong your IBD symptoms.

Your Gastroenterologist

A gastroenterologist is a medical doctor who has spent an extra three to four years training in the field of gastroenterology and hepatology. Our specialty is known affectionately as "guts and butts," so it includes diseases of the esophagus, stomach, liver, gallbladder, pancreas, small intestine, and large intestine (colon and rectum). A gastroenterologist is not a surgeon, so although this doctor performs procedures like colonoscopies, it is a surgeon who performs operations such as removing the gallbladder or draining abscesses. Not all gastroenterologists have a special interest in IBD; I urge you to find one who does.

Some gastroenterologists are particularly busy performing procedures. So, the bulk of your regular care may be from a specially trained NP or PA at the gastroenterologist's office who will discuss your case with a supervising physician. NPs and PAs write prescriptions, order

TABLE 2. Preventive Health Care Measures

Tuberculosis Test	Radiology
Vaccinations	DXA scan
Hepatitis A	Mammogram
Hepatitis B	Colonoscopy
Human papilloma virus	Postoperative
Influenza	Dysplasia surveillance
Pneumococcal	Laboratory Exams
Td/Tdap (tetanus)	Complete blood count
Mumps, measles, rubella	Liver function tests
Varicella/zoster	Creatinine
Annual Exams	B_{12}/folate/iron
Pap smear	25-Hydroxyvitamin D
Breast/prostate	Lipids/glucose
Blood pressure	
Ophthalmologic	
Skin cancer	

tests, offer referrals, and have their own office schedules. Some perform flexible sigmoidoscopies in locations that have only a few gastroenterologists. They cannot perform colonoscopies or other complex procedures or admit patients into the hospital. In general, NPs and PAs have more time to educate patients and can be more knowledgeable about living with IBD and the newest medications than many physicians.

Do You Need a GI Specialty Center?

Some of my patients have wondered if they need to be cared for at medical centers that have a special focus on IBD. I usually try to explain that there are different levels of "specialty" even within IBD. Those centers that see more than just a few IBD patients a week tend to be the places that run clinical trials, offer the most up-to-date therapies, and have the most experience with complicated cases. They also are a good resource for second opinions.

But this may require travel on your part and added financial pressures. Also, it's possible to feel overwhelmed in the setting of such a large institution, where you might be seen by several different physicians, some of whom are still in training, at different stages of your care. You might not know who your primary physician is, with so many attending your case. You may prefer to deal with one medical professional in a small office setting who works within smaller hospitals and doesn't do as much teaching or training. I encourage each of my patients to find what "fits" best to their personality, location, information needs, and other circumstances.

The Surgeon

In some areas, surgeons are more plentiful than gastroenterologists. Surgeons perform procedures like colonoscopy in addition to operations. Sometimes a patient is diagnosed with Crohn's disease after going to the doctor or hospital with what appeared to be appendicitis—and has never seen a gastroenterologist. Patients with ulcerative colitis who undergo a J pouch procedure may go back to their surgeon when they have difficulties with the surgical outcome and not necessarily to the gastroenterologist who took care of them when their colon was still intact. Because surgeons do not have specific training in the medical aspects of IBD, I believe they are your go-to professional when you need surgery but not for your general and IBD care.

The Hospitalist

Some practices have doctors who have specialized in the care of hospitalized patients. This "hospitalist" may make decisions regarding your care when you are hospitalized with a flare of IBD. The hospitalist works in conjunction with the health care provider whom you see as an outpatient. This doctor does not have a role in your care once you are discharged from the hospital, although you may have a significant relationship and develop a bond while you're going through some of the toughest days of living with IBD.

How to Get the Most from Your Health Care Visits

- Have an agenda with a list of issues/topics you want to discuss in order of priority—in case you don't get to all of them in a single visit.
- Bring someone else or a tape recorder with you or take notes, so that you don't lose any of the valuable information after you leave the office.
- Be realistic in your expectations. Your health care provider isn't able to cure you, nor does he or she have unlimited time to spend with you.
- Ask about ways to be proactive in your IBD self-management. Your daily efforts will pay off and make your visits positive experiences.
- Request copies of each test result after each visit. Keeping these records makes it easier to be aware of your condition and to share your information with additional or new health care providers.

6

Medications
for IBD

Although IBD is not curable, we can use medications to try to control the inflammation and alleviate your symptoms and prevent the long-term consequences and damage that can be caused by inflammation. There are no magic bullets or cures. Any entity that claims it can cure IBD is based on patient testimonials and not controlled clinical trials. A "clinical study" does not make a therapy legitimate, either. Therapies have to be tested in a controlled manner, either versus a placebo or in the same patients for a time using the drug and a time off of the drug, for comparison—that is the "controlled" part of the process. People with IBD can go into prolonged remission, but that is with continued use of medications and is not considered a cure. Medications are very important but cannot replace other good habits, such as getting enough sleep, and have to be taken in the appropriate manner to be effective.

What can medicines do? Some only help control symptoms, like antidiarrheals and pain medications, while others control inflammation, such as steroids. Therapies like azathioprine and the biologics can actually heal the lining—repair the inflammation so that it looks totally normal again. Table 3 at the end of this chapter summarizes all the common therapies used to treat IBD grouped by category. Below is a "treatment pyramid" showing the typical patterns for treatment choices (Figure 7). As your disease becomes more active or severe, the higher we climb on the pyramid.

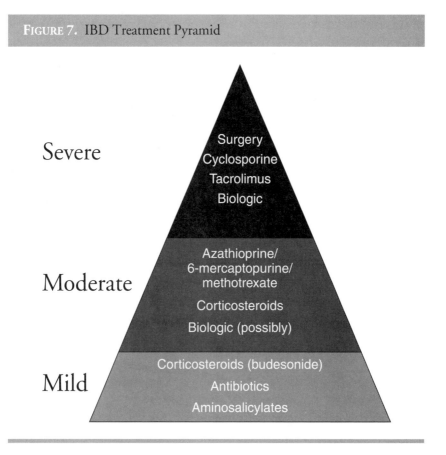

FIGURE 7. IBD Treatment Pyramid

Severe

Surgery
Cyclosporine
Tacrolimus
Biologic

Moderate

Azathioprine/
6-mercaptopurine/
methotrexate
Corticosteroids
Biologic (possibly)

Mild

Corticosteroids (budesonide)
Antibiotics
Aminosalicylates

Medications for IBD Inflammation

Aminosalicylates

This class of drugs works at the level of the lining of the gut. Aminosalicylates do not affect the immune system at all, and that is why they are considered the safest of the medications. The active ingredient of these preparations is 5-ASA (aminosalicylic acid), and they are considered to be anti-inflammatories. Although they are related to aspirin (salicylic acid) and the other pain relievers like ibuprofen and celecoxib (Celebrex), aminosalicylates are very distant relatives and have completely different methods of treating inflammation. How distant relatives are they? It is like comparing a Great Dane to a Chihuahua. Both are dogs that were bred long ago from a common ancestor and clearly share some characteristics, but they are not the same at all. For children taking aminosalicylates, there is no worry for Reye's syndrome, a condition that comes from aspirin use.

There are different forms of 5-ASA, namely mesalamine, balsalazide, olsalazine, and sulfasalazine (see Table 3 on page 80). The body breaks them all down to the same active ingredient: 5-ASA. They work by "mopping up" the proteins at the lining of the gut that are causing the inflammation. They do not inhibit the proteins from being made, but they do stop them from being able to work. The analogy I like to use is that these are mops that clean dirt from the floor. The mop does not stop the dirt from collecting; it just cleans up after the fact.

Remember Michael, the 31-year-old with ulcerative colitis? At diagnosis, Michael was started on a 5-ASA product that he took twice a day for his colitis. He noticed a difference in his symptoms within 2 weeks and then complete resolution of his symptoms by 8 weeks. This is the usual pattern, that some symptom relief is noted fairly quickly, particularly rectal bleeding. To feel back to normal takes a bit longer. You may recall that Michael thought that was the end of the therapy for his ulcerative colitis, so he stopped taking the medication. When his symptoms returned, he started 5-ASA therapy again, and it took a couple of more months before he felt "right" again.

Joann's symptoms of ulcerative colitis were a little more severe than Michael's. She was having many stools each day and even some that occurred in the middle of the night, about once a week. She required a higher dose of 5-ASA for her more moderately active disease. Her symptoms improved again after about 2 weeks, but it took at least 10 weeks for her to get rid of the diarrhea.

The 5-ASAs have FDA approval to treat active disease and maintain remission for ulcerative colitis.[33–43] Although many patients with Crohn's disease are prescribed these agents, the majority of the data suggests that they are no more effective than placebo unless the Crohn's disease is confined to the colon or, if in the small intestine, is very mild.[44, 45] However, they are very effective for ulcerative colitis and associated with very few side effects. In fact, long-term use has been associated with decreased risk of cancer.[46]

With this class of medicines, the thinking is, "more can be better." Some patients with more aggressive disease may need up to 4.8 grams of medicine a day, whereas others only need half that much. There is no increase in side effects with an increased dose, so if your disease requires more for relief of your symptoms, it is not an issue to use more.[47, 48] The exception to this is sulfasalazine, which does have more side effects the more you take, but is a very effective agent that also helps with joint pain (see Chapter 7 for more about IBD-associated joint pain). However, many are intolerant or allergic to the sulfa component, which is why the other sulfa-free agents were developed.

All of the agents in this class essentially work the same, so it is a matter of preference in terms of capsules or pills, amount per unit, and cost. All of the aminosalicylates can be taken twice a day, or even once a day if that's all you need. We used to recommend that they be taken three or four times a day, but with decades of use and further study, we have found that's not necessary.[49] There are subtle differences between the agents, just like differences between brands of peanut butter or toothpaste. Therefore, most of the time, which one you use is a matter of your own personal preference.

Occasionally, patients experience worsening symptoms on 5-ASA agents, usually within a few days of starting them. If your diarrhea and bleeding become worse when starting on any of these agents, it signals an allergic-type reaction to the medicine. You will have the same thing happen with any of the other agents of this class, so it doesn't help to switch from one to another. Because this is a reaction that cannot be reversed or overcome, you'll need to find alternatives to treat active disease.

For the majority who tolerate them and see a benefit, there are some rare side effects to watch for, including hair loss, headache, inflammation of the lining of the lungs or heart, inflammation of the pancreas, and kidney damage.[50] Specific to sulfasalazine, this agent can cause damage to the bone marrow. So, taking these medications requires some additional medical monitoring to ensure your safety.

Antibiotics

We use antibiotics to fight infections like abscesses and fistulas around the anal area that can develop in Crohn's disease. We also use them after an operation and in combination with other medications to treat active inflammation. It is common to use metronidazole (Flagyl) and ciprofloxacin when patients may have bacterial overgrowth in their small intestines as a result of narrowing or prior surgeries. These agents have activity against the kinds of bacteria commonly found in the GI tract. It is unclear, however, whether antibiotics really help in either Crohn's disease or ulcerative colitis when there are no abscesses to treat.[51, 52] We use rifaximin and tetracycline when a patient cannot tolerate or has become resistant to the more commonly used antibiotic agents.

If you have ulcerative colitis, in particular, you need to know about a certain bacterium that is normally found in the healthy gut called *Clostridium difficile.* Your gut naturally contains many different bacteria. When you take an antibiotic, it can wipe out certain kinds of bacteria, which can sometimes allow *C. difficile* to multiply and grow to much higher numbers than is normal. This bacterium produces a toxin that at high levels causes inflammation. Overgrowth of *C. difficile* is also common among residents of nursing homes or people who are hospitalized.

Unfortunately, with so many people using antibiotics, we are seeing *C. difficile* strains that are resistant to conventional treatment. People without any other risk factors, like recent antibiotic use, are getting *C. difficile* infections, and having IBD seems to make you even more susceptible than others to *C. difficile* infection, which can result in flares, hospitalizations, and even death.[53] The infection is diagnosed by testing stool for presence of the toxin and then treated with either metronidazole or vancomycin, which are antibiotics. If I suspect *C. difficile* infection is behind a bad flare of colitis symptoms, I often treat for it even before I have the results of the stool test. This bacterium travels as spores, which can live outside the body and on surfaces for up to 60 days. The best way to prevent and control *C. difficile* is with vigorous hand washing and by cleaning surfaces that have been in contact with stool with a bleach-based solution.

Steroids

Steroids have been the cornerstone of medication treatment for very active IBD.[54-56] They are inexpensive, work quickly, and can be given orally, intravenously, or rectally as suppositories or enemas. If your symptoms are severe, steroids can "turn them off" quickly, which is often just the break you need. Steroids work by essentially shutting down the entire immune system, which helps control the inflammatory reaction in the GI tract. Although this is an effective strategy for IBD symptoms, it comes with a big price to pay in terms of side effects.

Sharon, the 17-year-old with newly diagnosed Crohn's disease, was prescribed prednisone in the hospital emergency department when her CT scan showed Crohn's disease. Within a day, her pain was much improved and she was able to eat. Her diarrhea also got better within a couple more days. However, she developed acne and was unable to sleep due to feeling so "wired."

Tad, the man with disease in his jejunum, was also given prednisone after his diagnosis. However, his symptoms did not get better because they were being caused by a narrowed, scarred section of bowel without any active inflammation. Steroids will not help this kind of damaged bowel.

Whether you have ulcerative colitis or Crohn's disease, you need to consider steroid use very carefully. Keep in mind that a steroid is not a long-term therapy. Indefinite use of steroids leads to long-term side effects and essentially steroid-dependent IBD. So, when you and your doctor decide to start a course with a steroid, there should be a clear plan for going off of it—an "exit strategy."

The most common form of oral steroids used is prednisone in adults and methylprednisolone in children under age 16. A typical starting dose is 40 milligrams (mg) per day, given either once a day or, more likely, in divided doses. Divided doses allow for a more even level of steroid available throughout the day, rather than a lot of medicine in the morning and none by the end of the day. Some health care providers will give as much as 60 mg per day, but there is little evidence that the extra 20 mg is worth the extra side effects for most people.

Steroids are commonly used when someone is hospitalized for IBD. In the hospital, intravenous doses are given until the disease activity is controlled and then patients are transitioned to oral steroids. However, it is fairly common for patients to have problems after they are discharged from the hospital if they were transitioned too quickly from the intravenous to the oral steroids. It's important to do this properly. We need to have evidence that patients have a good chance to stay well on oral therapy, such as the ability to sleep through the night or manage their cramps without pain medications.

Immediate or short-term (up to about 6 weeks) side effects of steroids can include weight gain, mood swings, acne, hair loss, problems with blood flow to the larger joints, an increased risk for infections, increased appetite and energy level, and higher levels of blood glucose. Although having increased energy sounds positive, it can actually be in the form of anxiety and jitteriness, along with insomnia. In terms of mental health, steroid use tends to "make the highs higher and the lows lower," so a good mood can feel euphoric, and if you are sad, you may be tearful and even depressed.

Long-term (longer than 6 weeks) effects include thinning of the skin, easy bruising, osteoporosis, steroid-induced diabetes, hypertension, and cataracts. Because your body naturally makes about 5 to 7 mg of prednisone a day in the adrenal glands, taking steroids sends a message to your glands to shut down because they are not needed. That is why it is important to wean off of the steroids slowly and carefully, to allow your body to figure out it has to start calling on the adrenals again to provide prednisone. Patients who are weaned too quickly can go through withdrawal, which is characterized by lightheadedness, weakness, headache, joint pains, and sometimes fainting and loss of consciousness. People on steroids are more at risk for complications when they are in accidents or have surgery or get another illness. These are extra stresses to the body, and your body's normal reaction to such a stress is to increase the amount of steroids it produces. This ability is now diminished.

It is important to remember that, even years down the road, the effects of steroids can remain with you. Varicose veins, thin fragile veins, cataracts, and diabetes are just a few things that can happen well after steroids are stopped if you take them for a long period. Because everyone has a different threshold for sensitivity to steroids, the definition of "a long period" varies. But if you have been treated with 7 to 10 mg over four months, there would be adequate time to see the long-term effects.

Steroids come in enema form also, but studies suggest that the enemas made with aminosalicylates actually work better than steroids and have fewer side effects.[57–59] Side effects with enemas are not as frequent as with oral steroids, but because they are still absorbed into the bloodstream, steroids via enema should be limited to no longer than about 12 weeks.

As we learn more about alternatives to steroids, we are also finding that steroid use is associated with the worst outcome in patients.[60] But because steroids can work so quickly to provide relief in a dire situation, we tend to use them. However, the trend now is to avoid steroids altogether by using alternatives or beginning immunomodulator or biologic therapy early in IBD management, so the need for and the effects of steroid use are minimized. Steroids have not been shown to actually heal the intestinal lining, as have other medications, so this is another reason why we are becoming more hesitant to use them.

There is one steroid that helps in mild to moderate Crohn's disease without the typical steroid side effects. Budesonide (Entocort EC) can work just as well as prednisone for Crohn's disease of the terminal ileum and right side of the colon.[61–66] But unlike regular prednisone, it doesn't continue to circulate as long in the bloodstream. Once absorbed by the terminal ileum, close to 90% of the drug is removed from the circulation by the liver. This makes it an effective locally acting steroid but not so effective when your disease is spread over a larger area of the GI tract or you are having very active inflammation. If it is working for you, you might use budesonide for several months before you need to be weaned off of it. There are no controlled studies to show that oral budesonide can replace prednisone in treating ulcerative colitis, but in enema and suppository form it can be very helpful when combined with 5-ASA.[67] If this combination is right for you, your doctor may direct a pharmacy to make an enema or suppository for you to use (they are not available by regular prescription).

You need to avoid steroids if you have osteoporosis, an infection, uncontrolled diabetes, or a history of significant psychiatric side effects to steroids, such as psychosis or suicidal thoughts. Because there are other options, my advice is to work with your doctor to avoid or minimize the use of steroids in your IBD management.

Immunomodulators

6-Mercaptopurine and azathioprine. Originally developed to treat leukemia, immunomodulators (a form of immunosuppression) are a class of drugs that, at much lower doses, helps control the part of the immune system responsible for the uncontrolled inflammatory response the body is producing. 6-Mercaptopurine and azathioprine are the two immunomodulators most commonly used to treat ulcerative colitis and both the inflammatory and fistulizing types of Crohn's disease.[68–72] Because they suppress the actions of one part of the immune system, rather than the entire immune system as steroids do, and overall are safer than steroids, immunomodulators can help you avoid or stop using steroids. For this reason, we refer to them as *steroid sparing.*

Sharon, the young woman with Crohn's disease who got better on steroids, then needed something to control her disease instead of the steroids. In this situation, immunomodulators are the best choice. As her doses of steroids got smaller and smaller, she took an immunomodulator so that it built up slowly in her system. Within 3 months of starting 6-mercaptopurine (6-MP), Sharon was off steroids and feeling well.

There are some things to know about immunomodulators for IBD management. First, although they are effective, it takes anywhere from 3 to 6 months of use before the full benefit takes effect. So, you need to use something else for the short term.

Also, immunosuppressants have potential short- and long-term side effects, but when you and your doctor work together and you have proper monitoring, the results are very effective. I tend view the use of these drugs like the keys to a fancy sports car: put them in the hands of a novice 16-year-old driver, then it's likely there will be trouble, but in the right hands, you can have a high-performance machine.

The short-term adverse events, sometimes called allergies, include

- fever, as high as 103°
- rash
- joint pains
- pancreatitis, which is inflammation of the pancreas, the organ that secretes insulin and digestive enzymes

These tend to occur in the first 3 to 4 weeks of use in about 7% to 10% of all patients who use them. If any of these reactions occurs, it's not safe for you to stay on this type of medication. But you can get around the mild nausea that can occur by taking these medications at night or with food.

Another common side effect occurs when the drug does its job too well and actually decreases your white blood cell count, which makes you susceptible to infections and illnesses. A decreased white blood cell count is entirely reversible if the drug is temporarily stopped and restarted at a lower dose. Because you won't have any symptoms from a decreased white blood cell count, your health care provider will need to monitor for this on a regular basis with blood tests. In fact, there is a blood test that helps us know how efficiently you are able to metabolize azathioprine and 6-MP; note that azathioprine is broken down by the body and turned into 6-MP, so they are essentially the same drug. We do this test, called the *TMPT enzyme test*, prior to deciding on the dose to predict your risk for a decreased white blood cell count.

Immunomodulators can also cause slight damage to the liver, which is also monitored with blood tests. If damage to the liver does occur, it is reversible with stopping the drug or decreasing the dose.

But perhaps the most frightening long-term effect for my patients is the association of these drugs with the development of lymphoma, which is cancer of the lymph nodes.[73, 74] Here are two key points to keep in mind about this:

- the overall risk is still relatively low
- alternatives, like active disease or steroids, are associated with higher risks of poor outcomes, including death; using these drugs can actually lower that risk

Methotrexate. The other commonly used immunomodulator is methotrexate.[75–80] We adopted this drug to treat Crohn's disease from rheumatologists who use it to treat rheumatoid arthritis because, in addition to treating inflamed bowel, it is particularly helpful to those with painful, swollen joints. Although available in pill and shot form, it's usually given by injection because it is not well absorbed by the inflamed GI tract. Methotrexate is faster acting than 6-MP or azathioprine, inexpensive, and taken just once a week by self-injection.

On the down side, the methotrexate shot can cause flu-like symptoms that can last 24 hours. It competes with the body for folic acid, so you need to take folic acid supplements daily. As with the other immuno-modulators, you'll need blood tests to monitor liver function and blood counts for white cells. Although there is no increased risk for lymphoma, it does increase the risk of lung damage with long-term use, so we must also monitor for that. If you have other health issues that also put you at risk for liver damage, like diabetes, obesity, or excessive alcohol use, be particularly careful when considering using this drug. Overall, this is a very effective drug as long as you do the proper monitoring.[81]

Cyclosporine. Cyclosporine is another immunosuppressant used for severely active ulcerative colitis,[82–88] for fistulas,[89, 90] and for a skin condition associated with IBD called *pyoderma gangrenosum.*[91–93] It's an antirejection drug given to those who have received an organ transplant to inhibit possible organ rejection. However, suppression of this part of the immune system also appears to help those with IBD in certain situations.

Cyclosporine is given intravenously in the hospital for severely active ulcerative colitis and works over a matter of days. If you're not getting any benefit within 3 to 4 days, it is stopped. With the approval of Remicade for very active ulcerative colitis, cyclosporine has now fallen out of favor at some hospitals. Although effective, it can lead to abnormalities in blood potassium and magnesium levels, high blood pressure, and kidney damage. It is meant to be used for short periods (3 months or less) because of these side effects. It is also given intravenously to treat fistulas and pyoderma gangrenosum (there is more information about this skin condition in Chapter 7).

Tacrolimus. Tacrolimus is an immunosuppressant that is used in transplant patients and some patients with Crohn's disease.[94, 95] In particular, it helps those with fistulas that won't heal with other standard therapies. Tacrolimus comes in a cream form for topical use as well as in pill form. We use the cream to treat the skin condition pyoderma gangrenosum (see Chapter 7). Tacrolimus has the unpopular potential side effect of diarrhea—which is not very welcome in someone who already has or is prone to diarrhea. If you take it, your doctor will monitor the blood levels of the drug because kidney damage can occur when levels are too high.

Biologics

For those who cannot tolerate or don't respond to an immunomodulator, the coming of biologic therapy has been revolutionary. Biologics are in a new class of therapy, because they are not chemicals but proteins that are "grown" in a special factory. These proteins are antibodies that act to inhibit the activity of your body's specific immune system proteins that are causing inflammation.[96] One target is tumor necrosis factor (TNF), an inflammatory protein that is active in a variety of medical conditions. By blocking its activity, the body can heal.

At present, biologics are delivered via either intravenous or intramuscular injections because they are proteins, so stomach acid would break them down and render them inactive if given orally. Because antibodies have to be made by replicating the exact original antibody over and over, each biologic agent is patented. This is what makes these agents so expensive and why there will never be generic versions.

They work relatively quickly and can be used instead of steroids or to help you get off of steroids. But you can't just use it as needed. We have come to understand, with experience, that once you have introduced one of these agents, you have to continue to use it. Once you stop, your body forms its own antibody to the biologic agent that, via an allergic reaction, renders the medicine inactive. Here's how I explain this scenario: Suppose you have a relative who comes to stay with you for a while. At first you don't like them, but then you get used to their ways and a routine develops. Now let's say the relative leaves for a while, then comes back. Now you remember why you didn't like them in the first place and rally to get them to leave again. That's how your body deals with these kinds of therapies. Therefore, you have to stay on this therapy to keep it working. That's a big commitment, so I usually save biologics for people with more active, severe IBD.

The first biologic, infliximab (Remicade), has been on the market for more than 10 years and is given intravenously to treat Crohn's disease, either inflammatory or fistulizing, and ulcerative colitis.[97–109] It is engineered to be 75% human and 25% mouse. Since then, two more anti-TNF agents have become available. Adalimumab (Humira) is an injectable biologic that treats active Crohn's disease.[110–113] It is made from 100% human protein. Although you can give it to yourself and it's administered every other week, it is not any less expensive than Remicade due to the technology it takes to manufacture it. The other available biologic is certolizamab pegol (Cimzia), which is also injectable and given once a month, but unlike Humira, it is injected by either a health care professional, usually a nurse, or the patient. Cimzia also treats active Crohn's disease[114–118] and also is 100% human. We used to think that it mattered how much of a biologic is nonhuman, but it turns out that, because all of these proteins are foreign to you, your body has just as much chance of reacting to a medication that is part mouse as one that is all human.

I'm not convinced that any of the biologic agents are better than the others. Because the cost, effectiveness, and potential side effects are all comparable, the decision has to be up to you. When I am working with a patient who has active Crohn's disease to decide which one to begin, we discuss insurance coverage and that person's preferences.

I have some patients who like Remicade because it is given at an infusion center where health care professionals are available if there are any problems during or after the infusion. Also, some like to be able to take half a day off work or school to come and perhaps meet up with acquaintances who are also receiving infusions that day. I have had more than one romance develop among my patients as a result of meetings at Remicade infusions. Sometimes, just a chance to catch up on reading or watch a DVD is a plus. Other people like the convenience of giving themselves the shot of Humira every other week. And yet others cannot imagine giving themselves an injection, even though it is with a short, fine needle like that in an Epipen system, so they are more comfortable with the thought of a nurse coming to their home or going to their physician's office to receive the injection of Cimzia at their convenience once a month.

As I noted above, because the biologics are antibodies, your body can form its own antibody against the antibody. This is confusing, I know, but it results in an allergic or "hypersensitivity" reaction, or a loss of response. This is like walking into the bakery and at first smelling all the wonderful smells. But if you stay long enough, you get used to the smells and don't sense them any longer. In the case of Remicade, this leads to hives, shortness of breath and/or wheezing, and sometimes fever and chills during or one week after the infusion. You can also develop really bad joint pains and swelling, so it's easy to mistake the reaction for the flu. These reactions are different than the "allergic" reaction you can have the very first time you use a biologic. (In that instance, your body has an immediate reaction to the antibody by yet a different mechanism that does not require any prior exposure to the agent at all.) Premedication with an antihistamine and Tylenol, plus a one-time shot of steroids, can often prevent a hypersensitivity reaction. I do not automatically premedicate everyone, but some physicians do. We have not yet determined any differences in significant outcomes if you are premedicated from the start or not.

If you experience a reaction despite the premedications, especially if it's quite severe, then you are considered allergic to that agent. We can switch you to one of the other biologics, because being allergic to one agent doesn't mean that you will have a similar reaction to the others. With the injectable biologics, allergic reactions can happen at the injection site, where large hives, redness, and swelling can occur. However, sometimes the antibodies can develop and rather than give you an allergic reaction, it just makes the agent ineffective. In other words, despite your infusion or injection, you don't feel like you got any benefit at all. When this happens, I might try increasing the dose or decreasing the time between doses. But for some people, the agent stops working all together. One of the ways to avoid these possible reactions is to give these agents on a regular basis. If you take them on an irregular basis, you are much more likely to develop an allergic or immune reaction.[119, 120–121, 122] This is why it is so important to commit to the biologic once the decision has been made to use it to treat disease.

Remicade, Humira, and Cimzia are all associated with an increased risk of infections because they act by deactivating TNF, which is an important component of the immune system that fights off infections. These anti-TNF agents increase the risk for infections from bacteria, viruses, and certain kinds of fungi that are normally found in the air and are inhaled. They can reactivate tuberculosis if it is lying dormant in your body, so it's mandatory to undergo a TB test before starting this therapy. While blood monitoring is not required during therapy with these agents, we need to pay careful attention to any new symptoms that might suggest an infection.

The other risk associated with all biologic agents is lymphoma, which is cancer of the lymph nodes.[123–125] Note that I use the words "associated with" and not "caused by." It is still unclear to us why patients using biologics—for any condition, not just IBD—appear to have a higher rate of certain types of lymphoma than those with the same disease who are not on these agents or those in the normal population. We are following large registries of patients who are taking these agents to give us a better sense of what is being reported and to watch for changing trends. Based on our early experiences with these agents over the first decade of use, lymphoma appears to be a risk, and so for now it's important to note that lymphoma is more likely the longer biologics are used. How much more likely? If we agree that the risk of getting lymphoma in the normal population is about 2 in 10,000,[126] then using these agents doubles or triples your risk to about 4 to 6 in 10,000.

Another biologic introduced within the past few years is directed not toward TNF but to another protein that blocks cell movement and attachment to the lining of the gut.[127–129] Natalizumab (Tysabri) was first approved for multiple sclerosis but is now approved for use in active inflammatory Crohn's disease. It is considered a second-line therapy, meaning that we don't use it until someone has failed to receive benefit from at least one anti-TNF agent. It also helps reduce the use of steroids.

Tysabri has one side effect that unfortunately makes it somewhat unpopular: its association with a very serious infection that affects the brain.[130, 131] To date, there have been 11 cases of this infection in the more than 45,000 people treated with Tysabri. Progressive multifocal leukoencephalopathy (PML) is caused by a virus that almost all of us normally harbor in our bodies. It appears that the use of Tysabri can somehow activate this virus, which then attacks the brain. Because so many people carry this virus around in their bodies, it makes no sense to prescreen for it because there's no way to predict whether the virus will become active. PML is incurable and can lead to permanent disability and even death, but if caught early enough, it can potentially be treated with special techniques that wash the blood and system of the virus. Therefore, special precautions are in place to monitor everyone who is prescribed Tysabri. First, patients using Tysabri cannot be on any other immunosuppressants, and if they are on steroids, we must document a decreasing dose over time. If there is no response within 3 months, it is discontinued. Since its introduction in the United States for multiple sclerosis and Crohn's disease, there have been eight new cases of PML (all in people taking it for multiple sclerosis, not Crohn's disease) in addition to the three cases originally reported while the drug was in clinical trials. Based on the total number of cases of PML and the number of people who have received Tysabri therapy in total, the risk of PML infection is approximately 1 in 4,000.

Renee is a 27-year-old woman with a history of Crohn's disease involving more than 70% of her entire small intestine. She was on steroids for years at a time and had to have a hip replacement due to bone damage from her prolonged exposure to those drugs. Because most of her bowel is involved in the disease, surgery is not an option—she would not survive if all the disease was cut out. Renee was on Remicade for years, then stopped responding to it. She was switched to Humira, and then Cimzia, but lost response to those also. At that point, Renee's options included life-long intravenous feedings and bowel rest, Tysabri, experimental therapies, or referral for a small bowel transplant. She chose Tysabri and has been on it for close to a year now. She is doing well—well enough to get married! We closely watch Renee for any signs of nerve or brain infection, and she is happy with her decision.

Maybe the idea of using biologic agents sounds horrible and scary to you. I don't view biologics that way, and they have offered hope to many of my patients with very active Crohn's disease or ulcerative colitis who could not tolerate or lost response to the other medications we have available. Each one of the biologics has demonstrated its ability to decrease the risk of hospitalization, increase quality of life, and, overall, ease the burden of living with IBD by reducing disease activity and lengthening the time between flares.[132–135] There are studies showing that patients are willing to take risks more readily than doctors are if a therapy has a good chance of working, because the perceived benefit is higher than the perceived risk.[136, 137] Every treatment decision is a balancing act between benefit and risk, but then, most decisions are. Think about something as simple as deciding to get in the car and drive to the grocery store: does getting groceries outweigh the risk of getting harmed in a car accident? So many people with IBD had to suffer the use of steroids continuously until these biologic agents came along and improved their lives with IBD.

Thalidomide

Although not a biologic, thalidomide targets TNF and so can be used to treat Crohn's disease. Originally approved to ease the nausea of pregnancy, it was found to be associated with a serious type of birth defect that results in a baby born with no limbs (a condition called *phocomelia*) and was pulled from the market. It has made a comeback over the past years, however, because of its potent effects on inhibiting the growth of new blood vessels.[138–141] Its relative, lenalidomide, has also been used in a small study and is thought to have less significant side effects than thalidomide.[142] New blood vessels grow in response to inflammation and are thought to be involved with the progression of Crohn's disease. Stopping this process can treat the disease. Thalidomide is available only by prescription from doctors who are registered in a special program to help prevent the use in anyone who may become pregnant.

Medications and Older Folks

I want to add a special note for older people with IBD.[143] Because of the increasing number of medications that we take as we get older, be sure to make your doctor aware of all the medications you are taking because of their potential effect on IBD. For instance, if you have arthritis and coronary artery disease, you are probably taking NSAIDs and/or aspirin, which may precipitate a flare. Even over-the-counter NSAIDs can cause a flare when added to prescription medications.

Choosing which medications to use to treat IBD is made more difficult because older bodies do not break down and use medications in the way they once did. You may have become more sensitive to certain medications and need less or you may not absorb the medication as well (or at all) and need more of it or a different one. Also, it is very important to watch for side effects from interactions of different medications. Some people take so many medications that it is almost impossible to predict what the effect on their bodies will be.

Here is short list of the known effects of IBD medications on elderly people:

- Aminosalicylates are well tolerated.
- Azathioprine and 6-MP are also generally well tolerated, although given the slow onset of action, they are not much use if you are acutely ill with IBD. Also, the risk of lymphoma is higher because of advanced age.
- As with younger people, there is often an increased effect when oral and topical (suppositories and enemas) medications are combined. (It may be more difficult for older people with arthritis, for example, to use rectal therapies.)
- There is no reported difference in the efficacy or safety of Remicade in the elderly.
- Corticosteroids have a higher risk of serious complications. Side effects include osteoporosis, cataracts, glaucoma, diabetes, psychosis, depression, infections, electrolyte abnormalities, congestive heart failure, and high blood pressure. Some of these conditions, like the drug-induced diabetes, will go away after the patient stops taking the steroids, but some will continue to require treatment and even surgery, in the case of cataracts.

Table 3 provides many details on the medications we use to treat IBD. I provided this detailed information because I believe that it's vital for you to be well-informed about your medications. This will help you get the most benefit possible. If you have any questions about your medications, the doses, or the adverse (side) effects, please speak with your gastroenterologist.

TABLE 3. Medications Commonly Used to Treat the Inflammation of IBD

Name	Class	FDA IBD Indication	Common Uses	Dosing	Common Adverse Events	Special Considerations
Prednisone, methylprednisolone, hydrocortisone	Systemic corticosteroid	None	Moderate to severe UC, CD	1–2 mg/kg to a max of 40–60 mg orally per day	Weight gain, acne, mood changes, puffy face, increased appetite	Not for long-term use; patients doing well on steroids are not in true remission; may affect growth in children
Budesonide (Entocort EC)	Local-acting corticosteroid	Mild to moderate CD of terminal ileum and colon	Ileocecal CD	9 mg orally for 6 wks, 6 mg for 2 wks, then off	Same as prednisone but occurs less frequently	Safer than prednisone but not for long-term use; used also for collagenous colitis, microscopic colitis
Cortifoam, Cortenema, Proctofoam	Topical/rectal steroid	None	Proctitis, active left-sided symptoms	Rectal application once to twice daily	Weight gain, headache	Some systemic absorption
pH-controlled mesalamine (Asacol)	5-ASA	Mild to moderate UC	Colitis	2.4–4.8 g orally (400-mg tablets)	Headache, diarrhea, abdominal pain	3–7% have worsening of colitis

Medication	Class	Indication	Dose	Side effects	Notes
Time-released mesalamine (Pentasa)	5-ASA	Mild to moderate UC	Small and large bowel CD, UC	2–4 g orally (250-mg or 500-mg capsules)	Headache, diarrhea, abdominal pain	3–7% have worsening of colitis
MMX mesalamine (Lialda)	5-ASA	Mild to moderate UC	Colitis	2.4–4.8 g orally (1.2-g capsules)	Headache, diarrhea, abdominal pain	3–7% have worsening of colitis
Granular mesalamine (Apriso)	5-ASA	Maintenance of UC	Colitis	1.5 g orally (375-mg capsules)	Headache, diarrhea, abdominal pain	3–7% have worsening of colitis
Balsalazide (Colazal)	5-ASA	Mild to moderate UC	Colitis	6.75 g orally (750-mg capsules)	Headache, diarrhea, abdominal pain	3–7% have worsening of colitis
Olsalazine (Dipentum)	5-ASA	Maintenance of UC	UC	2–3 g orally (500-mg capsules)	Watery diarrhea	
Sulfasalazine (Azulfidine)	5-ASA	None	Colitis	3–6 g orally (500-mg capsules)	Rash, nausea, headache	Folic acid supplementation recommended
Mesalamine (Canasa)	Topical 5-ASA	Active ulcerative proctitis	Proctitis	1,000 mg rectally once or twice daily (1,000-mg suppository)	Bloating, gas	Can be used in combination with oral 5-ASA
Rowasa enema	Topical 5-ASA	Active mild to moderate distal ulcerative colitis, proctosigmoiditis or proctitis	Proctitis, left-sided colitis	4 g rectally at night (4-g enema)	Bloating, gas, incontinence	Often used in combination with oral 5-ASA

(continued)

TABLE 3. Medications Commonly Used to Treat the Inflammation of IBD (*Continued*)

Name	Class	FDA IBD Indication	Common Uses	Dosing	Common Adverse Events	Special Considerations
Azathioprine (Azasan, Imuran)	Immunomodulator	None	More commonly CD but also UC	2–2.5 mg/kg body weight orally (50, 75, 100 mg)	Low blood counts, pancreatitis, rash, fevers	Regular blood counts essential for monitoring
6-Mercaptopurine (Purinethol)	Immunomodulator	None	Commonly CD but also UC	1–1.5 mg/kg body weight orally (50-mg tablets)	Low blood counts, pancreatitis, rash, fevers	Regular blood counts essential for monitoring
Cyclosporine (Neoral, Sandimmune)	Immunomodulator	None	Severe UC and CD, fistulizing CD	2–4 mg/kg IV then 2× IV dose orally	Hypertension, headache, tremors, facial hair growth, low magnesium	Levels need to be monitored to avoid complications; Bactrim for prophylaxis of pneumonia
Methotrexate	Immunomodulator	None	CD	25-mg injection for 12 wks, then 15 mg maintenance	Mouth ulcers, liver damage, scarring of lungs	Folic acid supplementation recommended; absolutely not used in pregnancy

				Strength		
Tacrolimus (Protopic)	Topical ointment	None	Cutaneous, perineal, perianal CD, pyoderma gangrenosum	0.03–0.1%, apply to affected area once to twice daily	Itching, burning of skin	Minimal absorption, but levels should be monitored initially
Tacrolimus (Prograf)	Immunomodulator	None	Severe UC and CD, fistulizing CD	0.1–0.3 mg/kg orally twice daily	Nausea, heartburn, diarrhea, kidney damage	Levels must be monitored, risks may outweigh potential benefits
Thalidomide	Immunomodulator	Orphan use for CD	Moderate to severe CD	50–250 mg orally daily	Nerve damage, sedation	Never used in pregnancy
Ciprofloxacin	Antibiotic	None	Fistulizing and colonic CD	500–1,000 mg orally daily	Rash, headache, diarrhea	Interacts with nutritional supplements
Metronidazole (Flagyl)	Antibiotic	None	Fistulizing and colonic CD	500–1,000 mg orally daily	Potential interaction with alcohol, metallic taste, nerve damage	Long-term use often limited by nerve damage, dose reduction may decrease risk
Rifaximin (Xifaxin)	Antibiotic	None	Fistulizing and colonic CD	600–1,200 mg orally daily	Nausea, diarrhea, abdominal pain	Used for traveler's diarrhea

(continued)

TABLE 3. Medications Commonly Used to Treat the Inflammation of IBD (*Continued*)

Name	Class	FDA IBD Indication	Common Uses	Dosing	Common Adverse Events	Special Considerations
Infliximab (Remicade)	Biologic agent (anti-TNF)	Inflammatory and fistulizing CD, UC	CD, UC, pouchitis, joint and skin problems associated with IBD	5–10 mg/kg IV at 0, 2, 6 wks induction then every 8 wks for maintenance	Infusion reactions, delayed hypersensitivity, URI symptoms, other infections	TB test must be performed prior to initiating due to increased risk of TB; possible to develop either intolerance or nonresponse over time
Adalimumab (Humira)	Biologic agent (anti-TNF)	Inflammatory CD	Active CD	160 mg, 80 mg every other week induction, then 40 mg SQ every other week	Injection site reactions, infections	TB test must be performed prior to initiating due to increased risk of TB; possible to develop either intolerance or nonresponse over time

Certolizumab pegol (Cimzia)	Biologic agent (anti-TNF)	Inflammatory CD	Active CD	400 mg SQ wks 2, 4 then every 4 wks	Injection site reactions, infections	TB test must be performed prior to initiating due to increased risk of TB; possible to develop either intolerance or nonresponse over time
Natalizumab (Tysabri)	Biologic agent (anti-alpha 4 integrin)	Inflammatory CD	Active CD nonresponsive to other agents	300 mg IV every 4 wks		Viral brain infection (PML)

Medications for Specific IBD Symptoms

There are some therapies that we prescribe or recommend to specifically treat symptoms, rather than the underlying disease process, of IBD. Because coping with diarrhea and pain are part of living with IBD, anti-diarrheals and pain medications are the two types of agents that fall in this category the most often.

Antidiarrheals

There are several different antidiarrheals available, some over the counter and some by prescription. Loperamide (Imodium) comes in pill, capsule, and liquid form as well as in combination with anti-gas agents. Whether you buy it over the counter or by prescription, all have the same strength. Loperamide acts in two ways to stop diarrhea: it slows down the muscular activity of the gut and it strengthens the tone of the anal sphincter. Generally, doses are in the range of 2 to 16 mg a day. Diphenoxylate-atropine (Lomotil) is by prescription only and works differently than loperamide. This combination of two drugs slows down the contractions of the intestines. Recommended dose is 2 to 8 tablets per day.

The best way to take loperamide or diphenoxylate-atropine is before meals, because it's the meal that stimulates the GI tract to evacuate. If you take your pills after you eat or have a loose stool, it is too late already. If you have chronic diarrhea or frequent loose stools, you need to take either medication before the diarrhea for it to be most effective. Because these two medications work in different ways, they are some-times used in combination with each other or other antidiarrheals.

Tammy is age 45 and has had three surgeries for her Crohn's disease. She is on 6-MP with good results for her disease, but because of the sur-geries, she has chronic diarrhea. Tammy uses loperamide on a regular basis: two tablets each morning and evening, and sometimes one in the middle of the day, to control the number of stools she has. She has experimented over the years with how many pills she needs to take at a time and has figured out what works best for her.

Another antidiarrheal is cholestyramine (Colestid, Wellchol), a medicine that binds bile. More bile than normal can flow to the colon because of intestinal surgery or if you've had your gallbladder removed. Bile is a direct irritant to the colon wall and causes a watery diarrhea. Cholestyramine binds the extra bile to remove it, which results in firmer stools. It can be taken up to four times a day, depending on the amount of bile that is reaching the colon.

Tincture of opium also alleviates diarrhea by slowing the muscular activity of the intestines, so it's not used if you are prone to intestinal obstructions. It comes in drops that you add to water and drink several times a day. It causes drowsiness, and because it is a form of a controlled substance, it requires a written prescription that must be renewed each month. Also, it will turn your urine positive for illegal drugs. Tincture of opium is probably third or fourth on the list of drugs to try for diarrhea because of its side effects and because it's difficult to get because it is a regulated drug.

Codeine is a pain medication that also treats diarrhea. As a side effect of its pain-killing actions, it also slows down the motor contractions of the intestines. It is less habit-forming that other narcotics but is the third or fourth choice as an antidiarrheal because it is a controlled substance and will produce a positive drug test.

Occasionally, a patient will have a very high stoma output leading to dehydration. In this case, octreotide (Sandostatin) can be used. This is a form of a hormone that our body makes naturally to help slow down all the functions of the GI tract. Octreotide is a shot that is administered several times a day and is quite expensive, so I see it as a last resort.

One remedy for frequent diarrhea that gets a lot of positive press, as well as support from my patients, is coconut macaroons. Specifically, Archway brand macaroons appear to have antidiarrheal effects in those with Crohn's disease. One or two cookies in the morning, and many people are good to go for the day. There seems to be something special about the Archway brand—perhaps the specific combination of sugar and coconut oil—that gives it this property because people who eat homemade cookies or other brands of coconut macaroons do not seem to be able to get the same results. I tell my patients that if their dentists don't mind them eating coconut macaroons daily, then I don't mind them using this to avoid having diarrhea.

Pain Medications

The active symptoms of IBD are often painful, so you will need to know how to manage pain medications. The most important point is that pain medications are meant to be used for relatively short amounts of time because of their addictive nature.

Acetaminophen is the preferred over-the-counter pain medication because it does not upset the stomach like other pain relievers can. Use it for headaches and other pains as well as to fight fever. The other common class of over-the-counter pain medicines, like ibuprofen, naproxen, and aspirin, can all cause inflammation and ulceration of the stomach and small and large intestine and should be avoided if possible. Several studies suggest that regular use of ibuprofen-like medications (nonsteroidal anti-inflammatories, or NSAIDs) can increase the risk of active disease (a flare) as much as 30%.[144–146] These anti-inflammatories work differently than the anti-inflammatories used to treat ulcerative colitis and Crohn's disease. When absolutely needed, like after dental or orthopedic work, conservative use of NSAIDs, with food, for the shortest amount of time is recommended.

Another nonnarcotic pain medication is tramadol (Ultram), which is taken orally several times per day. Physicians prefer this over narcotics because it does not have as much addictive potential as narcotics and is safer than the NSAIDs bought over the counter or prescribed. Ketorolac (Toradol) is a pain medication commonly given in hospital emergency departments for acute pain. Because ketorolac has been associated with kidney damage specifically in patients with IBD, you need to avoid using it.

We use narcotics such as oxycodone, meperidine, and morphine when patients have severe pain from active disease. But we also need to treat the underlying cause of the pain, which is active inflammation.

Once the disease is under control, it's important to wean you off of the narcotics.

Many people with Crohn's disease experience pain even when there is no evidence of active disease. This can be caused by overactive nerve stimulation that has occurred over years of active disease affecting the bowel wall. This type of pain should be treated with nonnarcotic pain medications and other nonmedicinal interventions, sometimes in conjunction with a pain specialist.

For those with ulcerative colitis, note that narcotics can slow down the bowel enough to make a sick colon even worse. If you have very bad cramping, it's better for you to take antianxiety medications that can relax the bowel rather than slow it down. However, if you are having intense, sharp pain, this can be a sign of impending perforation, similar to what happens with appendicitis. This is a serious situation that requires immediate medical care.

Future Treatments

We continue doing research to learn more about the mechanisms of inflammation, which will eventually allow us to develop more kinds of therapies. There are currently several different pathways under investigation, along with technology that will allow bacteria to deliver healthy proteins directly to the intestine wall after ingestion. And, there are agents sometimes used as last-ditch efforts to control Crohn's disease and ulcerative colitis that have not been studied in large trials. In short, the work continues, and here's a very brief report.

Agents for Ulcerative Colitis

- Rosiglitizone, a diabetes drug that reduces insulin resistance, has been used in trials and shows promise for mild to moderate disease because of its anti-inflammatory effects.[147]
- Phosphatidylcholine, a common fatty component of membranes found naturally in the body, has been used to help

increase mucus production in the gut lining and shows some promise for mild to moderate colitis.[148]

- Alternate biologics that work on different pathways than TNF, such as vedolizumab and abatacept.[149]
- A procedure called apheresis, which is a type of dialysis used to cleanse the body of the cells that are producing the proteins causing inflammation, reduces disease activity in the Japanese but does not appear to work in Caucasians.[150–153]

Agents for Crohn's Disease

- Bowel rest and total parenteral nutrition, which is feeding by infusion directly into the bloodstream, has been shown to heal fistulas and stop inflammation.[154, 155] This is not a long-term solution, because prolonged nonuse of the GI tract results in other problems, such as infection and possible liver failure.
- In small trials in Japan, AST-120, a form of activated charcoal, has been shown to help heal perianal fistulas.[156] However, it is not available for everyday use, and its long-term effect is unknown.
- Growth hormone shots in conjunction with a special low-protein diet have been shown to improve Crohn's disease activity in a small number of patients.[157, 158] We don't understand how this combination worked or the long-term effects of giving growth hormone on inflammation, particularly in terms of the development of cancer. A recent preliminary trial in pediatrics has shown promise and hopefully will prompt further controlled trials.
- Because it's possible that IBD is caused by a faulty innate immune system, one tactic for controlling IBD might be to wipe out the immune system of a person with IBD and start fresh with one from new stem cells.[12, 159–161] Research being conducted at Northwestern University in Chicago is investigating this treatment strategy. For people who are nonresponsive to all other agents, stuck on steroids, not surgical candidates, and otherwise in relatively good shape, this may be an option. The procedure

involves first harvesting your own stem cells from the bone marrow. Then you receive chemotherapy and radiation to wipe out your current bone marrow. Next, your stem cells are injected to repopulate your bone marrow with new immune cells that hopefully will behave normally. After this procedure, patients are on immunosuppressant therapy to prevent rejection. The few people who have undergone this procedure have had good short-term success, but it's not known whether they will stay in remission over the long term. Obviously, it is time consuming, has a lot of potential side effects from each of the steps, and is very expensive.

- A particular substance known as a stimulating factor is given to cancer patients after chemotherapy because it stimulates the bone marrow to produce new cells to repopulate their bloodstream. Similar factors have been given to patients with Crohn's disease to try to "flood" the system with new, immature white blood cells that are not activated to cause inflammation.[162] This was shown to help decrease symptoms in small trials, but the long-term effect of continually stimulating the bone marrow is not known and is believed too dangerous.

- Naltrexone is an inhibitor of pain receptors throughout the body that has also been found to inhibit certain inflammation pathways.[163] While intriguing, there are some important reasons to be cautious: these data were from an uncontrolled study of fewer than 30 patients, it was a short-term study, and the dose used is not readily available at any pharmacy. But the results were positive enough that a larger trial is currently enrolling in Pennsylvania.

Clinical Trials

Maybe the medications that you've tried have not worked or maybe they stopped working. Maybe you are stuck on steroids and can't seem to get off them. Maybe you had side effects from certain therapies that prevented their continued use. These are all reasons to consider joining a clinical trial.

At any given time there are multiple trials underway at different research centers across the country. In the past 10 years, clinical trials have produced agents that are targeted and better at treating IBD, and more are in the pipeline. Think about it: none of the therapies that we now have to treat people with IBD would be available if it had not been for clinical trials.

Participating in a clinical trial offers several advantages:

- You are receiving cutting-edge therapy that is not otherwise available.
- The associated medical care is free of charge to you, and you may even receive some monetary compensation for your time and effort.
- You are helping to advance the science and care of IBD in general.
- It may be a chance to prove to yourself that you tried everything out there before undergoing surgery.

All clinical trials, regardless of their size or funding source, have to be listed on a special government Web site, www.clinicaltrials.gov. So this site is an excellent resource for learning about trials going on in your area or studying your particular clinical situation. Also, all clinical trials are first approved by ethics review boards not affiliated with the investigators or the pharmaceutical companies so that your rights are protected.

Staying on Your Medication

So, you are finally feeling great. That means you will want to ask, "Do I really need to take so much medicine? After all, it has been a while (thankfully) since I've had an IBD flare."

The answer is yes. It is very important to continue to take your maintenance medications. Here is a partial list of the reasons why:

- IBD is a chronic, incurable disease, just like diabetes. You wouldn't encourage your brother who has diabetes to stop taking his insulin just because he feels well.

- Inflammation in the digestive tract can be present even if you feel well, and it will get the better of you if you let it. Medications help to slow down the inflammatory process and promote healing, which ultimately leads to the decreased risk of potential future complications, like surgery or cancer.

- Even short-term discontinuation of medications, especially if you have required long courses of steroids in the past, leads to earlier disease relapse, compared to people who don't stop their therapy.[164]

- Not taking medications can lead to more aggressive flares, which may require steroid therapy, hospitalization, or surgery.[165]

- A long-term study performed at the University of Chicago showed that patients who were followed for two years had a *5-fold* increased risk for a disease flare of ulcerative colitis if they took less than 80% of their prescribed medication over that period.[166] Those patients who continued on their medications regularly were less likely to have to visit the doctor or have procedures and ultimately saved money.[167, 168]

- Two studies have shown that patients with Crohn's disease on long-term azathioprine therapy are at risk for a flare if they stop taking it, even when they have been well (flare free) for more than 5 years.

- Several studies have shown that taking 5-ASA medications over the long term may decrease your risk for the development of cancer.[46] It is unclear whether this protection is due to controlling inflammation or is a separate effect altogether.

Why would you stop something that is working for you? Well, perhaps your health care providers haven't done a good job of explaining what your medications do and why you need to continue using the ones that are working, so the reason behind all that effort is missing. Maybe the financial drain is overwhelming you. Maybe you think you can get by on a little less, so you are self-testing lower doses. Perhaps having IBD is a burden that you wish you would rather not have to deal with every day. Or you keep forgetting. Your reason may be unique and private.

It turns out that those patients who do not have a good support system are the ones most likely to stop taking their IBD medications.[169] This includes single people and young college students. Men, in particular, are susceptible to this behavior.

The way to avoid falling into this unhealthy trap is simple: get support from your health care team that will make things easier for you. Here are some ideas about how to do that.

- Ask questions! If you don't understand what a medication does or what you should expect from it, then you are less likely to take it.
- If you are having trouble paying for your medications, ask about generic formulations and patient assistance programs.
- Ask your health care provider whether there is a way for you to take your medicines twice or even once a day, rather than multiple times during the day.
- Keep small supplies of pills in several places so that when it is time to take them, you have some available. Taking them "later" often leads to skipped doses.
- Understand what to do if you miss a dose. Do you take it as soon as you remember, double up the next dose, or just wait until it's time for the next regular dose? What are the consequences if you miss too many doses?
- Be open and honest with your health care providers about everything you are taking or using. They may not like your choices, but at least they can then watch out for unwanted or unexpected side effects and interactions from the other substances.

Unconventional Therapies and Alternative Approaches

People with chronic diseases often look for answers to their problems beyond the help offered by their health care providers. It's natural to want to know if something else—a new compound or therapeutic approach—exists that appears to work for others in your situation and whether it can help you. Taking care of your IBD yourself can help you feel more control over a disease that often seems to be in charge! You may also want to avoid the feeling of being too passive a participant in your health care. The vast unlimited resource that is the Internet is one place to turn, as are practitioners of what is often called *complementary and alternative medicine* (CAM). "Complementary" means that it works in ways that fill the gap left by conventional treatment for a disease. "Alternative" means it is a different approach from conventional treatment.

Most individuals use CAM not as an exclusive choice or because of a dissatisfaction with or rejection of conventional medication but as a genuinely complementary approach, out of a willingness or eagerness to do whatever seems reasonable to them to improve their condition and maintain their health. Surveys in different countries have estimated CAM use among people with IBD to be 31% (Cork, Ireland), 47% (Berne, Switzerland), 57% (Winnipeg, Canada), and 69% (Los Angeles, California).[170–177] CAM therapies used by those with IBD fall into several categories:

- food/diet
- exercise
- mental therapy: meditation, prayer, relaxation techniques, biofeedback
- physical manipulation: acupuncture, acupressure, chiropractic, massage
- oral therapy: vitamins, herbals, probiotics, homeopathy

People with IBD have revealed that they most commonly use the types of CAM that are taken orally, with herbal remedies used by 45% in one survey, and homeopathy used by 52% of people surveyed in Switzerland but just 16% in Canada. Many have turned to chiropractic (used by 41%) or massage (23%) therapy. Also, mental therapies are used by others: prayer by 17% and relaxation techniques by 17%. If it feels good and appears to help, why not do it?

My primary concern is about your safety. I want my patients with IBD to be aware of common CAM approaches and knowledgeable about what information exists regarding their safety and how well they work. As with any medication, the doses, duration of use, type of preparation, and potential interactions are all critical factors that someone needs to evaluate and understand. There are few well-done studies to guide us in their use. Unfortunately, many types of CAM rely primarily on anecdotal reports spread through word of mouth or by Internet chat. Truly useful therapeutic approaches can be studied and shown to have positive results.

It is particularly important to inform your health care providers that you are using alternative approaches, especially anything you are taking orally. It's entirely possible that the agent you are ingesting is safe by itself, but when combined with other medications is not so safe. You may be tolerating an alternative supplement just fine but then you need to start another medication for a different condition, for instance an antidepressant or even just a short-term antibiotic. This can result in various problems, ranging from deactivation of the antibiotic to liver or kidney damage. Two therapies by themselves may be fine, but put them together and now it's not so fine. My example is peanut butter and tuna fish—separately they make fine sandwiches, but put them together and suddenly it is not such a fine sandwich.

You may not want to share information about what alternatives you are using with your health care providers because so many professionals discount the benefits of CAM. It's a judgment call, and our judgment is typically based on evidence. Our job as medical professionals is to do no harm, and it's possible to harm you if we prescribe or recommend agents without knowledge of *all* things you are taking. There are good data showing that significant or severe adverse events related to a conventional medication are also more highly associated with CAM use.[178]

My Thoughts on Certain CAM Therapies

Aloe is a popular homeopathic remedy believed by some to heal colitis. Unfortunately, the cells that line your colon are nothing like the cells that line your skin, and there is no evidence to show that this works. There are many forms of aloe, and some extracts are actually harmful to the colon cells. Some other extracts are indeed being tested in the laboratory for healing properties, but this research is still being done in rats and is not ready to be tested on humans. Because most of us cannot tell which extract(s) may be in the formulation that is purchased, I recommend that patients use this only for their skin and not their colitis.

One of the more common IBD symptoms that can persist, even between flares, is nausea. It can be due to a medication side effect or the disease itself, or sometimes we just don't know. Try ginger; for many, it works well. Drinking ginger ale can soothe nausea, and chewing on a piece of fresh ginger or chewing ginger gum or drinking ginger tea are all ways to relieve nausea and is cheaper and safer than most of the drugs we use to treat nausea. This is even safe to use during pregnancy and for small children.

Fish oil (as omega-3 fatty acids) has been shown to be helpful in treating mild to moderate Crohn's disease and ulcerative colitis.[179–186] In these studies, it took 2 grams of one of the formulations available in Europe, which are much stronger than what we have in the United States, to treat active disease. You would need to eat about 12 pounds of fish a week to get that much omega-3. In addition, larger trials have failed to show any benefit for maintenance. So, use the formulations available here for your heart health but not as your sole treatment for Crohn's disease.

Curcumin, which is the ingredient in the spice turmeric, has anti-inflammatory properties. In small trials, it has been found to help maintain remission from flares but so far has not been shown to control active disease.[187, 188]

Maybe you have heard about "worm therapy" for IBD. Researchers in Iowa hypothesized that, because people in less industrialized nations do not get IBD, turning on the part of the immune system that fights parasites might turn off the part of the immune system that is overactive in IBD.[189, 190] They studied patients who were given the unhatched eggs of pig whipworm to ingest, which appeared to help with both ulcerative colitis and Crohn's disease and resulted in steroid use reduction and healing of the colon lining. Pig whipworm was chosen because it is not a known parasite in humans and not thought to hatch and cause disease in the human body. Several problems arose, however: some of the worms actually hatched and were seen during the colonoscopy, the FDA had an issue with doctors giving people worms to treat disease without its knowledge and approval, and the pig farmers became upset that they were not getting paid enough. Now, worm therapy is only available over the Internet from foreign countries. There are other parasites being studied. In Mexico, for instance, certain hookworms are implanted under the skin in the arm to incite the same sort of reaction to try to shut off the overactive part of the immune system. Although the theory behind these interventions appears valid, and the before and after pictures are compelling, I do not personally offer eggs to my patients nor inject hookworms under their skin.

For therapies or agents that my patients want to take (a partial list of some of these are in Table 4), I review them to see if there is any known association with adverse events and then explain that there may not be enough reliable information to show that they are helpful at all. Why spend money on something that has no data to back it up as effective? This is only a partial list, because the true number of CAM therapies people have tried is too large to list here. To sort through the many alternative therapies and supplements available, consult the Physicians Desk Reference of Herbals, Supplements, and Alternative Therapies (www.pdrhealth.com/drugs/altmed/altmed-a-z.aspx; medical professionals use the regular PDR to research existing conventional medications) to learn what is known about ones of interest to you. If the attraction of these remedies is that they are "natural," which we often think of as synonymous with being benign or free of side effects, remember that you wouldn't sit in a patch of poison ivy or play with jellyfish even though those are 100% natural. Use your head!

Probiotics

Probiotic therapy is potentially very useful in IBD.[191–196] Probiotics are the "good bacteria" that normally live in your GI tract and serve to help

TABLE 4. Partial List of Alternative Therapeutics Used to Treat IBD

Oral Therapies

Vitamin supplements

Herbal supplements

   Aloe vera

   Cats claw

   Soy-derived isoflavones

   Green tea

   Ginseng

   Slippery elm

   Boswellia serrata

   Calendula

   Chamomile

   Bach Flower Remedies

   Curcumin

Eggs of pig whipworm

Alternative Medical Systems

Homeopathy

Naturopathy

Ayurveda

Traditional Chinese medicine

Probiotics/Prebiotics

Nissle 1917

Saccharomyces boulardii

VSL#3

PB8

Homeostatic Soil Organisms/Primal Defense

Diet

Specific Carbohydrate Diet

Low-carbohydrate diet

Rice water diet

Physical Therapy/Exercise

Chiropractic/osteopathy

Feldenkrais

Aerobic exercise

Acupressure

Acupuncture

Reiki therapy

Therapeutic touch

Hypnosis

Mind-Body Interventions

Relaxation techniques

Prayer

Meditation

Distant healing (others sending compassionate thoughts about you via telepathic means) with the last stages of digestion and colon health. It is believed that in IBD the natural balance of good bacteria is disrupted, and thus should be replenished. There are millions of strains of bacteria in the human colon, and it's hard to know which ones are the most important. However, we know about some that have anti-inflammatory properties. Acidophilus, lactobacillus, and bifidobacterium species are examples of some of these.

There are literally hundreds of probiotic formulas available, some with just one strain and others with multiple strains. Just as one perfume is not right for everyone, there is not a one-size-fits-all solution for probiotics. Sometimes you have to try several formulations before you find one that seems to help. Probiotics sold as supplements in health food stores contain 10^9 to 10^{10} (1 to 10 billion) organisms per dose. While seemingly a large amount, one gram of stool contains 1×10^{12} (one trillion) bacteria.

I never discourage my patients from trying probiotics. Here are some points to keep in mind.

- Probiotics can be of help, but they should not be your sole therapy for IBD.
- For many people, probiotics improve the symptoms of bloating, gas, and some of the cramping and can help with irregularity.
- A probiotic is capable of giving you GI symptoms, depending on how it reacts with your individual system. Do your homework about which one to use and be clear about your goals.
- Because probiotics are bacteria, they have to be ingested live or else they are useless. They are protected from stomach acid by the outer coating of the capsule they come in or because of their natural defenses. Make sure the brand you buy has an expiration date and has been through some sort of quality control, as evidenced by a batch number on the box.
- Products can range from generic single species per capsule to combination capsules. There are products that are marketed by pharmaceutical companies that do have to abide by the rigors of quality control. Some examples include Align, Flora-Stor, Flora-Q, and VSL#3.

- You must take probiotics on a regular basis, or their effects wear off. If you can't use them consistently, don't bother at all.
- Probiotics do not cure or prevent disease. If you feel well, you can't feel any better with their use.

One particularly promising bacterium to keep an eye on is *E. coli* Nissle. There are at least six trials that have compared probiotics with this strain of bacterium to 5-ASA agents or placebo in people with either Crohn's disease or ulcerative colitis.[197–201] What they've learned is that these particular probiotics are as good as 5-ASA in maintaining remission—but they do not improve the symptoms of active disease.

A prebiotic, as opposed to a probiotic, is a food ingredient that provides a selective stimulation of growth or activity of beneficial native bacteria. In other words, you would ingest a specific food that selectively enhances the growth of specific bacteria. Prebiotics are now being looked at as potential alternatives to traditional therapies. However, the particular species and dose, as with any medicine, is critical.

7

IBD Affects More than Your Gut

W hen the gastrointestinal tract is not healthy, as in inflammatory bowel disease, the effects can appear in almost every part of the body.[202]

Eyes

Two eye conditions are associated in particular with having IBD. Fortunately, they are relatively uncommon, occurring in less than 5% of people with IBD. The first is uveitis, which is inflammation of the uvea, the entire middle layer of the eye. The uvea consists of three structures: the iris, the ciliary body, and the choroid.

The second condition is iritis, an inflammation of just one part of the uvea, the iris. The iris regulates the amount of light entering the eye by closing the pupil when there is too much bright light.

Either of these conditions will cause a painful, red eye and some blurred vision. Usually, only one eye is affected, rather than both. It is typical for one of these eye conditions to occur when the gut is also experiencing active inflammation. Only an ophthalmologist can diagnose uveitis or iritis, not an optometrist. Because it is so painful, these are both very serious conditions that have to be treated right away with eye drops that control inflammation.

Note that it's possible for you to develop other eye conditions that are actually side effects from IBD medications. The most common are cataracts caused by steroids and "pink eye," which happens more frequently when you are on immune suppressants because they interfere with your ability to fight common infections.

Liver

There are two liver diseases that may occur in people with IBD. One is known as *primary sclerosing cholangitis* (PSC), in which the walls of the bile ducts both inside and outside of the liver become inflamed (cholangitis). This eventually leads to damage and narrowing of the bile ducts, which are the passageways that carry bile from the liver. Chronic inflammation in the bile ducts can eventually lead to cirrhosis (severe liver scarring) and its complications, including liver failure and liver cancer. PSC is usually discovered when blood tests suggest an abnormality in liver enzymes. Otherwise, there are generally no symptoms until the disease has progressed. Diagnosis involves either an MRI of the liver and bile ducts (MRCP) or, preferably, endoscopy that specifically can inject contrast into the bile ducts to look for signs of the disease, such as strictures or narrowing of the bile ducts (endoscopic retrograde cholangiopancreatoscopy or ERCP), and sometimes a liver biopsy.

The severity of PSC, unlike the eye conditions, does not parallel the severity of IBD. The inflammation of IBD can be under control and the bile ducts inside and outside the liver can be actively inflamed, or vice versa. About 5% of people with IBD develop PSC. However, sometimes PSC is found first. It turns out that about 90% of those with

PSC have some sort of underlying IBD. We do not understand why the inflammation that occurs in this part of the body does not respond to anti-inflammatory therapies like the colon can.

We don't have an effective treatment for PSC or a way to prevent it or predict who might get it. Some doctors use a bile salt called *ursodiol* to help control the inflammation. Although ursodiol can improve the liver enzyme elevations and liver inflammation and damage in some people, it is not known whether this medication is effective in stopping the progression of this disease. The nature of PSC is variable: some people never experience any symptoms but clearly have abnormalities on imaging studies or blood tests and others have progressive PSC that does such damage that we need to consider a liver transplant.

The other liver disease associated with IBD is called *autoimmune hepatitis*. In this condition, the immune system begins to attack the liver, causing inflammation and damage. This is similar to what happens in the GI tract in IBD. The spectrum of symptoms of autoimmune hepatitis can range from none at all to liver damage bad enough to lead to cirrhosis and the need for a liver transplant. Autoimmune hepatitis is treated with medications that control inflammation, typically a combination of steroids and azathioprine. If someone has both conditions, then the same medication can treat both conditions.

The liver can also be harmed by IBD medications, including azathioprine, 6-MP, and methotrexate and, in rare instances, by sulfasalazine or infliximab. If you have a hepatitis B infection, you should not receive biologic therapy (those therapies made from antibodies rather than chemicals) as these can make the hepatitis infection worse. Also, using too much acetaminophen, which is commonly used to control the pain of Crohn's disease, can damage the liver if dosages greater than 4 grams are used in a 24-hour period, or if smaller doses are used in combination with alcohol.

Gallstones that form in the gallbladder, where bile from the liver is stored, are more common in people with Crohn's disease, as well as in patients requiring prolonged intravenous feeding (total parenteral nutrition, TPN). TPN can also, over the long term, cause fat to be deposited in the liver, resulting in liver damage. It is important to mention this here because TPN can serve as therapy for Crohn's disease, particularly in those with a large amount of inflammation in the small intestine or large fistulas involving the bowel and skin. TPN can also serve as supportive care to provide calories and nutrition to those with Crohn's disease who cannot take in adequate calories or nutrients on their own.

Kidneys

People with Crohn's disease are more susceptible to developing kidney stones. This is because Crohn's harms the ability of the body to get rid of excess oxalate, a nutrient found in lots of foods. When patients have diarrhea or inflammation, the body loses calcium. Calcium is what binds oxalate in the colon. When there is not enough calcium, then the oxalate is free to be absorbed back into the bloodstream. Then it is deposited in the kidneys because it has nowhere else to go. As the oxalate builds up, it forms stones. (Note that if you've had your colon removed, you're not at risk for oxalate stones.) The stones may travel out of the kidney with urine, damaging the urinary tract and causing bleeding and pain. You may be familiar with someone who has passed a kidney stone. The pain it causes is compared to childbirth and occurs all of a sudden on one side of the back. Stones may be found on CT scan or even on plain X-rays. Treatment for stones includes a lot of oral and intravenous fluid to flush the stone through the system. Sometimes, a urologist has to go up into the bladder with a special scope and extract a stone that is stuck. Some patients can have stones broken up with ultrasound sonic waves. Treatment with extra calcium supplements helps to prevent oxalate from being reabsorbed and is one of the simplest and best treatments.

Crohn's disease and ulcerative colitis have been associated with certain autoimmune kidney diseases, but this is very rare. In Crohn's disease, inflammation from the surrounding colon and intestine can cause a connection (fistula) to form between the bladder and the intestines. If this happens, you can pass gas and sometimes even stool when urinating. Surgery to repair the abnormal connection is the most effective solution.

Some of the medications that are used to treat IBD can potentially harm kidney function.[203] In particular, 5-ASA medications (see Chapter 6) can cause kidney damage that is called "idiosyncratic," which means there is no rhyme or reason to the damage and can occur at any time and at any dose. Even though this is relatively rare, if you use 5-ASA therapy, your doctor will monitor your kidney function with blood tests on a regular basis, usually every 6 to 12 months.

Bones

Osteoporosis is a condition, usually associated with older age, in which the bones become abnormally thin and brittle. Having osteoporosis increases the risk of fracturing bones in the wrist, ribs, spine, and hips. These breaks can occur with a minor injury that wouldn't hurt a strong bone.

Bones can also break due to osteomalacia, but this condition is different from osteoporosis or osteopenia. In osteomalacia, bones are weakened by nutritional deficiencies rather than by thinning due to calcium loss. Osteomalacia can be reversed if the reason behind it is identified and corrected.

More than 5 million Americans have osteoporosis, and 1.5 million fractures occur every year due to osteoporosis. Another 21 million Americans have an early stage of bone thinning called *osteopenia.* Studies show that people with IBD, especially those with Crohn's disease, are at increased risk for osteopenia and eventually osteoporosis. Some estimates suggest that osteoporosis occurs in one in seven people with Crohn's disease and that nearly half of all those with Crohn's have osteopenia.[204]

The most important risk factors for osteoporosis in the general population—older age, being female, and low body mass index—are still the most important predictors of osteoporosis for those with IBD. But here are some reasons why the rate of osteoporosis is higher than normal in IBD.

- Corticosteroids like prednisone have powerful effects on bone metabolism. In fact, decreased bone density and increased fracture risk may occur within a few months of starting steroids. Even low-dose prednisone (5 mg daily) use is associated with fracture risk.

■ Immunomodulators such as cyclosporine and methotrexate may reduce bone density slightly.

■ IBD itself, especially Crohn's disease, may be a risk factor. Low bone densities have been noted in newly diagnosed patients, even before they have been treated with corticosteroids. It's possible that the higher levels of proteins associated with inflammation have negative effects on bone formation and speed bone loss.

■ When Crohn's disease involves the small intestine or there has been removal (resection) of the small intestine, you may have decreased ability to absorb calcium and vitamin D, which are essential for strong bones.

■ Many people with IBD have low body mass index. Being small is an independent risk factor for osteoporosis.

■ Cigarette smoking is a risk factor for osteoporosis, and many people with Crohn's disease have a history of or currently smoke.

When you have IBD, you are 15% to 45% more likely than the general population to develop an osteoporotic fracture, especially in the hip, spine, wrist, or ribs.[205] In most, but not all, studies, this fracture risk is slightly higher if your IBD is Crohn's disease rather than ulcerative colitis. Those with IBD who are most at risk for fracture are post-menopausal women, those with low body mass index, and those receiving steroids. Other risk factors include a history of heavy smoking, steroid treatment for at least 3 months at a time, or prior fractures.

To monitor this risk, talk to your doctor about a dual-energy X-ray absorptiometry (DEXA) scan. The results of a DEXA scan are usually given as a T-score. The T-score indicates how much different your bone density is from the general population. Osteopenia is diagnosed when the T-score falls between −1.0 and −2.5 and osteoporosis is when the T-score is below −2.5.

You and your doctor can find ways to manage IBD-associated osteo-porosis and reduce your risk of fractures. Talk with your doctor about which choices would work for you:

■ Make healthy lifestyle changes, such as daily physical activity and stopping smoking.

- Take in at least 1,200 mg of calcium every day. This can be a combination of dairy foods and calcium carbonate or calcium citrate supplements.

- Daily, take in 400 to 800 IU of vitamin D. If tests indicate you are already low on vitamin D, you might need even more than this amount.

- If your IBD maintenance depends on using steroids, talk with your doctor about options for getting off steroids and using medications such as azathioprine, 6-mercaptopurine, methotrexate, and biologics for control.

- If you are postmenopausal, hormone replacement therapy helps preserve bone density. Selective estrogen receptor modulators, such as raloxifene (Evista), may increase bone density and reduce fracture risk but must be balanced by understanding your risk of breast cancer.

- Bisphosphonates block bone loss that occurs when calcium is taken from bones for other uses in the body. Two oral bisphosphonates, alendronate (Fosamax) and risedronate (Actonel), can be administered either on a daily or weekly basis. Both medications have been shown to increase back and neck bone density and reduce back and hip fractures for both post-menopausal and glucocorticoid-induced osteoporosis.[206, 207] In addition, risedronate prevents bone loss in patients receiving cor-ticosteroids. However, some gastrointestinal side effects, includ-ing inflammation of the esophagus, may occasionally occur with either medication, making it necessary to try other treatments.

- Pamidronate (Aredia) given intravenously every 3 to 6 months has been used by some physicians to deliver bisphosphonates for those who cannot tolerate the oral preparations. Another intravenous bisphosphonate, zoledronic acid (Zometa), is given once a year.

- Nasal salmon calcitonin spray (Miacalcin) can effectively improve bone density and reduce fracture in the lower back, in women who are more than 5 years postmenopausal in particular. Calcitonin is a hormone important for bone health, and extracts from salmon are an easy source.

Preventing bone loss and bone fracture are very important goals for your IBD self-management.

Joints

When your gut is sick, it can make your joints hurt, too. Aching or pain in the joints in IBD is called *arthralgia.* This is different from *arthritis,* which is inflammation in a joint that over time damages the joint. There is no damage to the joints with the arthralgias associated with IBD. This arthralgia can occur in large or smaller joints of the body—hands, knees, and ankles—and usually the pain parallels the IBD activity in the gut. This pain can move from one joint to another, so you may have painful ankles that over time feel better but then have pain in a hip during another flare.

Arthralgias can also occur during steroid withdrawal, but this pain lasts only a few days with a decreasing dose of steroid. Painful joints can also be a result of azathioprine use and will also go away if you stop this medicine. We treat arthralgias by treating your active gut symptoms, and certain medications like sulfasalazine, methotrexate, and the anti-TNF agents can help the joints just as much as the gut (see Chapter 6).

There are two arthritic conditions in which there is destruction of the joint and bone. Ankylosing spondylitis and sacroileitis are back and hip (large joint) conditions that cause hip and back pain. We can find the abnormalities with an X-ray. These arthritic conditions have their own course and do not parallel inflammation in the gut. We treat them with medications similar to those used for rheumatoid arthritis. Sometimes rheumatoid arthritis and IBD occur together, but this combination is rarely the reason for joint pains.

In addition to causing osteoporosis, steroid use can damage joints. Steroids can cause a condition called *avascular necrosis* (AVN) in which the blood vessel that feeds the center of the bone dies. This creates joint pain and eventually destroys the joint.

Hair, Teeth, and Nails

Hair and nails are the parts of the body that are the last to get nutrition, so if you are sick, these can become unhealthy rather quickly. Hair thinning or hair loss can occur because of iron deficiency, stress caused by a delayed reaction to a serious flare even months after the flare is under control, and ongoing active disease. Drugs associated with hair loss include steroids, high doses of 5-ASA drugs, azathioprine, and methotrexate. Healthy nails depend on good nutrition. Vitamin and mineral deficiencies as well as active disease can cause delayed nail growth, brittle or easily broken nails, and nail discoloration.

Gum and tooth disease and poor oral hygiene can be a result of Crohn's disease because of ongoing inflammation in the gums, poor nutrition, or steroid use. It is also a side effect of smoking. Chronic vomiting can cause dental erosion from exposure to excessive amounts of stomach acid.

Skin

Two skin rashes are typically associated with having IBD. Erythema nodosum is a painful condition in which red nodules appear on the shins and ankles. About 15% of people with IBD develop this condition but it occurs in several other autoimmune conditions in addition to IBD. Erythema nodosum can even occur before any signs or symptoms of IBD show up. This skin condition parallels the activity of the GI tract. Treat the inflammation in the gut, and the skin gets better. Erythema nodosum starts off looking like a bruise but then gets redder and more painful, sometimes so painful that it's hard to walk. This is such a well-known skin condition that, generally, your doctor will not need a biopsy to make this diagnosis. It can sometimes be confused with Sweet's disease, which is another skin condition characterized by itchy red bumps but mostly on the upper body. Sweet's disease is another autoimmune condition, and although rare in those with IBD, it also tends to parallel the gut activity and is treated in the same way that the gut is treated.

The second skin condition is called *pyoderma gangrenosum,* which occurs in about 5% of those with IBD. It usually affects the legs but can also occur on the arm or around a skin opening (stoma). We do not fully understand why this skin condition happens more often in people with IBD. It starts off as a little bump that can look like a bug bite, but it gets bigger and bigger, particularly if you pick at it. The more you pick, the bigger the bump gets. Over time, the bump turns into an ulcer-like crater, which is very painful. Any manipulation of the area, such as taking a biopsy, actually makes it worse. This skin condition does not parallel the inflammation in the gut and runs its own course. Without treatment, it will continue to get worse, and you can develop multiple ulcers. If you catch this while the bump is small, sometimes a prescription skin cream will clear it up (tacrolimus, Protopic).[208] Otherwise, we use drugs that are also used to treat the gut, such as steroids, azathioprine, and anti-TNF agents. The ulcers usually leave a scar even when healed.

Some of the IBD medications affect the skin. You can have steroid-induced skin thinning, which results in easy bruising and unattractive stretch marks (striae). Steroids also cause or worsen acne. Methotrexate use is associated with skin nodules that resemble erythema nodosum. This is very rare but if you notice skin changes while on methotrexate you should mention this to your health care provider. The nodules will eventually go away if you stop the methotrexate, but your doctor needs to advise you on this adjustment to your therapy.

Conditions that Parallel GI Tract Inflammation	Conditions that Do Not Parallel GI Tract Inflammation
Iritis, uveitis	Autoimmune hepatitis
Arthralgias	Primary sclerosing cholangitis
Erythema nodosum	Ankylosing spondylitis, sacroileitis
Sweet's disease	Pyoderma gangrenosum

8

The IBD-Cancer Connection

Colon cancer, properly known as *colorectal cancer* (CRC), occurs in about 33 in 100,000 people in the United States.[209] Having IBD increases your risk for CRC twofold over the normal population, to about 60 in 100,000. Although scary, CRC is actually a relatively rare complication of IBD. Even so, because there is a connection, it's vital to accept the extra vigilance involved in monitoring for it. CRC can be prevented, and self-management is the key.

Most cases of CRC can be traced to a colon polyp, an inward bulge of the colon lining, becoming cancerous. We believe that CRC in IBD arises from precancerous *dysplasia*. Unlike the easy-to-identify polyps in people without IBD, dysplasia in IBD may occur in the flat lining of the colon. This is more difficult to see during a colonoscopy. Therefore, screening for it requires random biopsies throughout the colon in order to identify it.

The Risk of Colorectal Cancer

Your specific risk for CRC depends on how much damage is occurring in your colon and how long the damage has gone on.[210] Most studies have focused on CRC in individuals with ulcerative colitis, but we know that those with Crohn's disease involving the colon (Crohn's colitis) are also at increased risk. The risk increases as the duration of IBD increases, from approximately 2% after 10 years of disease to approximately 20% by 30 years of disease.

Known risk factors for dysplasia and CRC in ulcerative colitis and Crohn's colitis include some things that you have no control over: how long you've had IBD, how severe or extensive your disease is, and a family history of CRC (independent of a family history of IBD).[211, 212] It appears that being of a younger age at diagnosis also increases your risk. Another risk factor that is beyond your control is having primary sclerosing cholangitis (PSC), which is inflammation and scarring of the bile duct system in the liver. It is unclear why having this liver condition makes a person more susceptible to colon cancer, as other liver diseases do not increase the risk at all.

There are two risk factors that you do have control over, and properly managing them appears to offer promise in lowering your risk. The first is the degree of inflammation of the bowel, which can be controlled by proper medical care and self-management. The other is a condition called "backwash ileitis," in which the small intestine next to the ileocecal valve is exposed to inflammatory "backwash" through the ileocecal valve, which can be controlled by medications for the colitis.[213]

Preventing CRC

Most CRC in IBD can be prevented if both you and your health care team understand your individualized risk and follow published guidelines about CRC surveillance. The first step is to determine your risk based on the risk factors, as outlined above. Your age weighs heavily in your overall risk, given the increased risk of random colon cancer with advancing age.

The guidelines of many health societies, including the American Cancer Association, the American Gastroenterological Association, the American Society for Gastrointestinal Endoscopy, and the American College of Gastroenterology, recommend that you have surveillance colonoscopy with random biopsies after 8 to 10 years of IBD and that you repeat this every 1 to 3 years, depending on the findings. The random biopsies look for flat dysplasia, and you need additional biopsies of polyps, strictures, or masses. However, if you have PSC, this surveillance needs to begin at IBD diagnosis and be repeated each year.[214] Although we don't yet know why, those with PSC show a faster rate of polyp growth and cancer growth than others with IBD.

This may seem like a lot of effort, unpleasant preparation, and expense, but it can save your life. We can find precancerous dysplasia and get rid of it. Untreated, low-grade dysplasia can progress to high-grade dysplasia before becoming CRC.[215] If CRC has already developed, we can find it at an earlier stage where the chance of curing it is excellent. If CRC is not found, it can become invasive cancer, which is much harder to cure. The studies show that those who undergo surveillance colonoscopy and who develop CRC are more likely to have it discovered in its very early stages and decrease their risk of death from cancer significantly over those who are not enrolled in a surveillance program. In addition to periodic colonoscopy, you can also reduce your cancer risk by managing your disease so you can avoid flares. And we are getting better all the time at identifying dysplasia using magnifying colonoscopes, special stains of the colonic mucosa, and stool DNA markers.

Dealing with Dysplasia

There are several stages of dysplasia as it develops toward actual cancer. Low-grade dysplasia (LGD) occurs first. This can revert back to normal tissue, stay constant, or progress to high-grade dysplasia (HGD). Recent work has shown that, if it is not removed, in just 5 years LGD may progress to a higher grade or to cancer in at least half of those who have it.

We do not yet understand all the factors that determine which direction LGD will take, but we agree that having continued active inflammation is a risk factor for dysplasia and cancer.

Dysplasia is further classified by how many places it is found in the colon. If found in only one site, it is termed *unifocal,* and if found in multiple places, then it is called *multifocal.* We manage multifocal dysplasia much more aggressively than we do unifocal, because the chances of having dysplasia that was missed or of having it progress to cancer is much higher in multifocal dysplasia than in unifocal.

If your colonoscopy reveals dysplasia, your next step is to have your biopsies read by a second pathologist, particularly one who is an expert in the field. The gastroenterologist who did your biopsies can send your slides for the consultation without you having to travel yourself. If they agree with the reading of dysplasia, then talk with your physician about a referral to an IBD specialty center. It's important to discuss your options with professionals who treat IBD complications like CRC every day. The decision about what to do is highly individualized based on your health history, family history of polyps and cancer, your other medical conditions, and your personal preferences. You will need to consider and decide on whether to have surgery or frequent follow-up colonoscopies with specialized techniques to detect abnormal cells.

Eloise was age 55 when I started caring for her. She had a long history of Crohn's disease of the colon and would come in regularly for her colonoscopies. On one of her scopes, I detected a very small bump right inside her rectum—easily missed if her prep had not been as good or if I had not been thorough. I biopsied the bump, and the report came back that it was a very early cancer. Because it was at this very early stage, and because the traditional approach meant Eloise would lose her colon and have a permanent colostomy bag, we opted for more specialized tissue removal plus increased surveillance with more frequent colonoscopies. This is not an option for everyone, but fortunately the tumor could be removed completely via the colonoscope, without surgery. Three years later, we found another area of cancer, and this time there was no doubt that the colon had to come out. Although Eloise had to have a permanent stoma, she was grateful for the three years we were able to postpone that operation, and even more grateful that we saved her life by finding the second cancer early.

If the finding is HGD, most experts agree that, unless you are a poor candidate for surgery due to your age or other health conditions, you will probably need to have your colon removed. This is because HGD brings with it an almost 40% increased likelihood that cancer is already present somewhere in the colon. Sometimes, when the dysplasia is found in a polyp, removal of the polyp and regular follow-up colonoscopies (approximately every 6 months) is enough to keep you safe. Again, the decision about what to do when dysplasia is found depends on a lot of factors, and a second opinion is always worthwhile in this situation, especially if your colitis is under control and the recommendation is for surgery. It is important to have a frank discussion about your risks, with the emphasis being that CRC is curable in its earliest stages.

Using Medications to Prevent CRC

A number of medications appear to prevent the development of dysplasia and CRC in people with long-standing colitis. Folic acid, as a 1-mg supplement a day, has been shown to decrease the risk of dysplasia in ulcerative colitis.[216] Adequate folic acid intake is not difficult to achieve in the United States because it is a common additive in food and is found in almost all multivitamins.

The gallstone dissolution agent ursodeoxycholic acid (URSO) is used to treat other conditions of the bile ducts within the liver but also has been shown to prevent dysplasia and cancer in patients with IBD and PSC at doses of 300 mg twice daily.[217, 218] So this agent is now recommended independent of its therapeutic benefits for PSC alone. We don't know whether URSO is helpful in individuals with IBD who don't have PSC.

The mainstay of therapy for inflammation in ulcerative colitis, 5-ASA, has an emerging role in preventing dysplasia and CRC in chronic ulcerative colitis.[46] In several studies, using 5-ASA at doses of 1.2 gram per day or greater reduced the risk of cancer by 72% to 80%. Although more research is needed, consider that 5-ASA not only reverses inflammation in ulcerative colitis and maintains remission of inflammation but also may protect against CRC.

Other Types of Cancer .

Lymphoma

Lymphoma is cancer of the lymphocytes (the T and B cells), the white blood cells that make up the lymph nodes. There are two major kinds, Hodgkins and non-Hodgkins, depending on what the cells look like under the microscope and their genetic makeup. Among Americans, the risk of developing lymphoma is age dependent: the rate is 2 to 3 per 100,000 of those between the ages of 19 and 25 and rises to 39 to 54 per 100,000 after the age of 60. There are many different risk factors that have been described, including infection with the bacteria *H. pylori,* famous as the culprit behind the common stomach ulcer; exposure to certain pesticides; and having certain autoimmune diseases like rheumatoid arthritis, Sjogren's syndrome, and perhaps IBD. Some studies refute any increased risk in IBD, but most investigators believe that the risk is indeed increased. This is because of data from a study following patients with IBD in France. In the study, patients who used medications that suppress the immune system, such as azathioprine and 6-mercaptopurine and the biologic agents used to treat IBD, were more likely to develop lymphoma over time.[219] This increased risk was between two and four times higher than the baseline risk. Because risk of lymphoma increases steadily with age, it is important for you to consider this connection as you get older. Keep in mind that most clinicians believe that the benefits derived from controlling active IBD symptoms with these medications far outweigh the risk for development of lymphoma, and so we continue to use these medications routinely to treat IBD, as well as other autoimmune conditions.

There is a type of lymphoma that is seen in younger people, predominantly males, that is associated specifically with use of immunosuppressant drugs. Historically, this type of cancer was seen with azathioprine use, but recently a number of patients on Remicade and azathioprine together have been diagnosed.[220–222] This is a particularly aggressive type of lymphoma of the T cells called *hepatosplenic T cell lymphoma,* to distinguish it from the B cells that most lymphomas comprise. Because it is made of T cells rather than B cells, this lymphoma does not respond well to known chemotherapy agents and can be fatal. Before we began using Remicade in children, this tumor was only seen in those who were taking azathioprine. But as its use in children with IBD rose, so did the number of these lymphomas. Because this type of lymphoma is most often seen in people under the age of 20, we now have special warnings against the use of Remicade in younger patients and have ceased using combinations of drugs in younger patients. Also, most younger patients have been taken off other immunosuppressant medications because of this risk. It's not clear whether the use of other biologic agents results in the same risk, but for now, it is recommended that Remicade be used by itself to treat either Crohn's disease or ulcerative colitis for these younger patients.

The symptoms of lymphoma can be very nonspecific, and sometimes we discover it only because a CT scan was done that showed abnormality in the size of the lymph nodes. Symptoms can include anemia, fatigue, unexplained weight loss, night sweats, and fever. Because these symptoms describe a lot of other conditions, a workup for lymphoma includes a physical exam of the body to feel for any enlarged lymph glands in the neck area, armpits, and groin. Otherwise, some kind of X-ray is needed; blood tests may not necessarily be helpful. People with IBD have response rates similar to the rest of the population in terms of chemotherapy, and usually the disease goes into remission because of the assault caused by the chemotherapy on the immune cells of the entire body.

Ryan had long-standing Crohn's disease of the small intestine. While in for his routine visit, we noted that he had lost a few pounds. Ryan was not that big to begin with, so I asked him if he had noticed the weight loss. He had not. He said he was feeling a bit more tired but thought it was work related. At our next visit six months later, Ryan had lost more weight. He admitted that he had been having some sweating at night, which he had never had in the past. An X-ray showed a new stricture in the middle of his small intestine, and he went to surgery.

The surgery revealed that the narrowing was from lymphoma of the small intestine, rather than scar tissue from his Crohn's disease. After a regimen of chemotherapy, he felt great and had more energy, and his weight returned to normal.

Cholangiocarcinoma

Cholangiocarcinoma is cancer of the bile ducts. It is a very rare cancer and usually associated with conditions that cause inflammation and scarring of the bile duct system, as in primary sclerosing cholangitis (PSC; see also Chapter 7). Thus, if you have IBD and PSC, you need to be monitored on a regular basis with blood tests that screen for changes in the level of liver enzymes, particularly one called *alkaline phosphatase,* that may signal an abnormality with the bile ducts. Usually there are no symptoms before the diagnosis is made, because tests are done based on abnormal blood results. If a tumor grows such that it affects the flow of bile, you would develop jaundice. Bile that cannot flow properly also can deposit in the skin and causes diffuse itching. Unexplained weight loss and vague abdominal pain can also be symptoms. Diagnosis is made by a combination of imaging and sampling of cells from the bile duct system, collected usually during an endoscopic procedure (ERCP). Cholangiocarcinoma is very difficult to treat, because it usually is not found until it is fairly far advanced. Some people have been treated with liver transplant if the cancer has not spread outside the liver.

Rare Tumors

It's possible to develop cancer inside a long-standing fistula. This is very rare and is reported in the literature on a case-by-case basis. Also, a fistula in the perianal region can develop cancer, but it would not necessarily be visible until it produced symptoms. Therefore, if you have a fistula that doesn't heal for more than 10 to 15 years, it's important to have it monitored for any change in its size or appearance.

Another rare cancer that is associated with Crohn's disease is cancer of the small intestine.[223, 224] Long-standing inflammation and scarring of that area can produce abnormal cells that reproduce and turn into cancer, similar to CRC. If you have Crohn's disease of the small intestine, you need regular monitoring with X-rays for changes that could signal either lymphoma of the small bowel or a primary cancer of the small bowel. Changes that are noted include irregular narrowings (strictures) or thickening of the bowel wall. There is no standard protocol for how often these tests should occur, because exposure to radiation without any symptoms is a risk unto itself. The increasing availability of MR technology will certainly help reduce this risk.

9

When You Need Surgery for IBD

Surgery is an important therapeutic tool in the management of IBD. In fact, surgery can offer advantages over medicines in several situations, so don't necessarily consider it to be a "last resort." Sometimes someone is so sick that surgery is best done before other complications set in, like perforation or infection. My job as a gastroenterologist is to make patients better, and sometimes that is with an operation. Take a few steps back and look at the big picture: Have you worked your way through all your medication options without success? Is continuing your medication therapy just leading to more complications without the promise of improving your health? This is a situation to discuss with your physician.

Let's say you have ulcerative colitis that has not gotten better despite many efforts at medical therapy or only responds to high doses of steroids. I would want you to consider what you are achieving by walking around with a sick colon. A colon is not an essential organ. Essential organs are those without which you cannot live—brain, heart, lungs, kidneys, and liver. It is certainly a convenient organ to have, but when it is sick and you have little or no control over when it evacuates, it can make for a very burdensome life. Almost without exception, patients who have undergone surgical removal of a sick colon later ask me, "Why did I wait so long?" They never realized how much their life was being compromised by carrying around such a burden. Once the colon has been removed, your disease is essentially cured because in ulcerative colitis only the colon is involved.

For Crohn's disease, the story is different. One of the reasons that health care providers may hesitate to recommend surgery for Crohn's disease is because the disease will come back. It recurs at the place where the diseased bowel was removed and the two ends were reconnected. Within 3 years of an operation to remove diseased or narrowed intestine, more than 80% of patients have recurrence of their disease.[225] This is not a reason to avoid surgery if it will make you better; it simply means that it's important to create a well-thought-out treatment plan for after the operation. After surgery, the focus is on preventing a recurrence of the disease. Researchers are working on treatment strategies that will hopefully decrease this recurrence rate, but at this point we still cannot fully stop it from coming back. It is important to remember, however, that there are different definitions of "recurrence." Some people consider recurrence when they can see it with an endoscope or on an X-ray even though the patient has no symptoms; others say it is when a patient has symptoms; and still others say the disease has recurred when the patient needs another operation.

An upside to surgery is that medications you may have tried without much success before surgery might just work better for you after the surgery. Essentially you now have a "clean slate" for them to maintain rather than asking them to fight an uphill battle against inflammation.

Common Types of Surgery

The most common type of surgery is a *resection*. This means that a part of the bowel is removed. This is done for disease that does not respond to medicines, when cancer is found, or when the intestine has developed a hole or perforation. Surgeons are learning new techniques to minimize the amount of bowel that is removed and to prevent complications and prolonged hospital stays. The decision on how much bowel is removed is based on information gathered from X-rays, colonoscopies, biopsies, and also visualization of the bowel at the time of the operation when the surgeon can actually see and feel whether bowel is healthy or not. More and more surgeons can perform resections or even remove the entire colon laparoscopically, which results in smaller surgical scars, less postoperative pain, and shorter hospital stays.

John had been having abdominal pain for a couple of days, much worse than the twinges he had experienced over the past 10 or so years. He thought it was probably something he had eaten. It was the kind of pain he would often get if he ate a big salad or an ear of corn. But when the pain continued to get worse, and he started running a fever that would come and go, he went to the hospital emergency department. A CT scan showed scarring of the last few inches of his small intestine, but so much scarring that there was hardly any opening left for passage of food into the colon. The intestine above this narrowing was stretched (dilated), and there was food sitting in the enlarged portion. John quickly found himself in surgery to have the strictured piece of bowel removed. When inspected, it was found to be chronically inflamed with Crohn's disease. After surgery, John had no further episodes of pain after eating and realized that he had been putting up with the discomfort when there was actually something wrong.

Stricturoplasty, where the bowel is stretched open with a balloon or surgically stretched, is another technique to limit the amount of bowel removed. This is done in the instance of a stricture, or narrowing, of the intestine. If the surgeon can stretch it open and make it usable, it does not need to be removed. This is sort of like when a heart specialist does an angioplasty: the blood vessel around the heart is stretched open or cleared of the cholesterol buildup, and this prevents the need for bypass surgery. How long you stay in the hospital after surgery depends on what kind of procedure you had and how sick you were going into the operation.

Because we are trying to perfect transplants for the vital organs—kidney, liver, lung, and heart—there's not much research into colon transplants, and it won't be a standard therapy any time soon. Perhaps stem cell research may someday enable us to grow new colons, but I don't know of any stem cell research labs working on that at present.

The small intestine is, on the other hand, an essential organ for sustaining life, and transplantation of the small intestine is possible. This procedure is limited to only a few centers around the United States because there are many complications related to the procedure and organs are difficult to come by. Only those people with Crohn's disease who have had so many operations that there is hardly any bowel left, who have so many strictures that the bowel is essentially unusable, whose disease does not respond to any known medical therapy, or who have already developed complications from intravenous feedings and can no longer be on them are candidates for small bowel transplant. This is rare, and I have yet to refer anyone with Crohn's disease to a center for small bowel transplant.

Medical Definitions Used in IBD Surgery

Colectomy: removal of the colon.

Dysplasia: precancer; describes cells that have become abnormal and are likely to become cancerous.

Ileal pouch anal anastomosis: the standard operation offered to patients with ulcerative colitis requiring removal of the colon.

"J" pouch: the shape of the pouch that is constructed from small intestine used in an ileal pouch procedure.

Ostomy: any external opening from an organ to the skin.

Resection: removal of a piece of bowel.

Stricturoplasty: a procedure where a stricture is stretched open with a balloon or other means and not removed.

TPN: total parenteral nutrition, which is nutritional support supplied via a large vein.

Thrombosis: blood clot.

Toxic megacolon: a complication of ulcerative colitis in which the colon becomes extremely dilated and the person is very sick.

Surgery for Ulcerative Colitis

In ulcerative colitis, surgery involves taking out the colon. It is important to understand that the *entire* colon comes out, even if some of the colon is normal. I get asked all the time, "How come I need to have normal colon taken out if it is just the last part of my colon that is diseased?" Many years ago, surgeons tried to take out only the affected parts and sew healthy colon to the anus. This did not work, and patients ended up with multiple surgeries with the same ultimate outcome. The example I give is this: imagine trying to sew a handkerchief (healthy bowel) around the top of a soda bottle (the anal canal). The kerchief is flexible and can be "scrunched up" but the top of the soda bottle is fixed and stiff. The anal canal is like that within the body. Unless you are Martha Stewart, it would be very difficult to figure out how to neatly cinch together all the edges of the kerchief around the top of the bottle without having uneven edges. Then, imagine trying to fill the kerchief with water and have it flow into the bottle without leaking. Impossible! That is what it is like if you try to attach the right side of the colon and the anal canal.

Having a colectomy done is a big, important decision to make. Sometimes, there are reasons when colon surgery is absolutely the right direction to take. These are if you have:

- medically resistant disease
- toxic megacolon
- cancer or precancer (dysplasia)
- perforation (a hole in the colon)
- hemorrhage (bleeding that does not stop)

If you have run out of options with medications without getting healthier, colon removal can help you. In rare cases, the colon remains so inflamed that the wall becomes dangerously thin and the colon stops working very well, which causes material to collect that leads to distension and fever and is very painful. This condition is aptly titled *toxic megacolon*, because the colon has become a fully filled, inflamed poison center that requires immediate removal. Because the walls are not strong, the colon can perforate. Luckily, this doesn't occur too often anymore because physicians are better at determining when a colon is so sick that it risks becoming a toxic megacolon. Aggressive medical treatment is the way to prevent both toxic megacolon and hemorrhage from developing.

Colon Removal

In the old days, when we took a sick colon out, patients had to live with an external bag (ostomy). Today, the standard procedure for colon removal is an ileal pouch anal anastomosis (IPAA), also known as a *J pouch procedure*. When complete, this procedure allows you to avoid an ostomy bag and to eventually move your bowels pretty much like anyone else, where you have the sensation of needing to go and then sitting on the toilet to evacuate. There are only a few reasons why you might not be a candidate for this procedure, so get a second opinion if you are told that you can't have one. Some reasons include a deformed anal canal that would not tolerate a connection, a small intestine that is too short to allow for a pouch to be built and then connected to the anal canal, an unhealthy ileum, or a history of many surgeries of the abdomen that would make it difficult for a surgeon to safely construct a pouch and attach it to the anal canal.

The J pouch procedure is done in stages to allow for proper healing at each step. The first stage is removal of the colon, with the rectum left in place. The surgeon creates a temporary stoma (opening in the abdominal wall) for a bag (ileostomy) that will empty the digested food coming from the small intestine. Because this is a relatively simple and straightforward surgery, this can be done by a general surgeon. What this means is that, if you need to have this surgery done on an emergency basis, you do not have to have a permanent bag just because there is no J pouch specialist available at the time.

The next stages, however, require a surgeon experienced in J pouch procedures. In stage two, the surgeon constructs a pouch from the end of your own small intestine. This pouch will serve as storage for digested food, and it no longer serves to digest or process food like it did before. Then, in stage three, the surgeon connects the pouch to the anal canal

FIGURE 8. Typical J Pouch

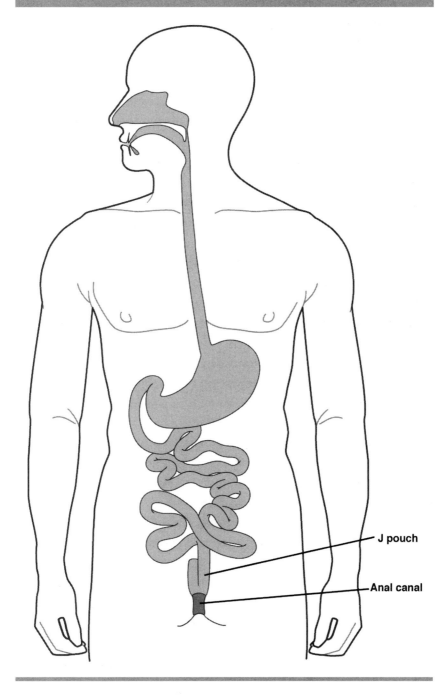

of the rectum and removes the stoma. Sometimes these procedures can be combined into the same surgery, but the same two steps are involved. Doing it in steps allows for healing and produces the best long-term outcomes. The goal is for you to develop fecal continence, which means better quality of life, more like a person without IBD. This entire process takes anywhere from 4 to 12 months and totally depends on your health at the time of the first surgery; how much steroid you are taking at the time of your surgery or the total amount you've taken over the course of your IBD, which may delay wound healing; and personal situations that make timing of the surgeries feasible, such as job considerations, family obligations, and vacation plans.

The J pouch functions as a reservoir, which enables you to evacuate stool as your schedule allows. You do go more often than most people— six to seven times per day—but with control. The pouch is constructed of your small intestine and connected directly to the anal canal, which is why it is so important to make sure that the small intestine (terminal ileum) is normal before proceeding. If there is evidence of significant inflammation in the small intestine, this may eliminate your chances for having this surgery.

Issues with Pouches

Pouches have a long life, and most never require a follow-up surgery to make changes. It is important on an intermittent basis to scope the pouch to make sure that it is still normal. Because there is usually a tiny amount of rectal tissue that is left behind as the surgeon attaches the pouch to the anal canal, bleeding can occur from this tissue.[226] Because there is a cuff of rectal tissue remaining, when it becomes inflamed, we call this "cuffitis." This is usually treated with anti-inflammatory suppositories.[227] Only in severe cases does a surgeon have to revise the pouch and remove that cuff of tissue. This does not necessarily sacrifice the pouch itself, but it can alter the function of the pouch (more bowel movements and some urgency).

Short-term complications of J pouch surgery include leaking from the connection between the small intestine and the anal canal, diarrhea and anal leakage, and obstruction from swelling or scar tissue.[228] Leaking at the connection would give you pain and fevers and blood tests would signal that you had an infection. We would see fluid within the pelvis outside the pouch on CT scan. If this occurs, the surgeon would most likely detach the pouch temporarily to allow for more healing. Diarrhea and leakage usually get better with time and adjustment to the pouch. Swelling of the intestine from the surgery itself or scar tissue (adhesions) can cause the bowel to kink and cause an obstruction; signs of this are nausea, vomiting, abdominal pain, and lack of output from the pouch. This is treated with bowel rest and time. However, if the kinking persists over days, you need another operation to cut away the scar tissue. This is not a sign that the disease has come back but a reaction of your body to the procedure itself.

J pouch procedures are done on an individual basis after someone reaches the age of 65 to 70. There is no significant difference in the frequency of leaks at the suture sites than in younger patients. But because an elderly person faces the possibility of more cardiac and respiratory complications and a longer postoperative hospital stay, this has to be taken into consideration when deciding on whether to have a J pouch (a multistep procedure) or a permanent ileostomy.

Longer-term complications usually are inflammation of the pouch (pouchitis) or stricturing of the anal canal. About half of all people with a J pouch get at least one bout of pouchitis; it's easily treated with antibiotics. Symptoms include frequency, urgency, cramps, and bleeding. In a few people, pouchitis becomes more difficult to treat, and antibiotics are required long term to keep the pouch healthy. One study that found starting certain probiotics (a formulation called VSL#3) right after surgery prevents pouchitis, but because not everyone gets pouchitis, this is not a standard treatment at present.[229, 230] Probiotics are not harmful unless taken in really large amounts, which can increase the risk for infections by fungus, but are expensive and require regular, daily use, so it's really your decision whether to use them.

Another cause of "pouchitis" can actually turn out to be Crohn's disease.[231] As often as we try to make sure that the diagnosis is ulcerative colitis before surgery, sometimes it just isn't 100% possible. Chronic problems with the pouch, particularly if there is inflammation of the small intestine above the pouch, suggests Crohn's disease. All is not lost if this is the case, because this can be treated medically, with therapies for Crohn's disease. In some instances, people known to have Crohn's disease of the colon but with a normal small intestine have colectomies and then have pouches built, with the understanding that if Crohn's develops in the pouch or small intestine, he or she will need to start therapy for Crohn's disease.

Talking about the complications of a pouch may be off-putting, but studies have shown that people with pouches have just as good, if not better, quality of life as those with an intact but sick colon.[232, 233] They don't have to worry about daily medications that may be suppressing their immune system; they can go to work and participate in activities without having to know where a washroom is all the time. With the advent of laparoscopic techniques, surgical scars are smaller and cosmetic issues are minimal.

There are a few exceptions to the standard J pouch procedure. The small intestine is sometimes attached to the rectum and no internal pouch or stoma is created. This procedure is done by only a few surgeons in the country and for very special circumstances, such as when a young woman is planning on pregnancy in the future (there is information on fertility in Chapter 13). Avoiding removing the rectum prevents scar tissue from forming in the pelvis, scar tissue being the culprit of fertility issues later in women who have undergone a J pouch procedure.

Surgery for Crohn's Disease

Roughly 80% of people with Crohn's disease have an operation at some point to manage their disease. It may have been exploratory surgery for what was thought to be appendicitis but turned out to be a diagnosis of Crohn's disease. It's common in Crohn's to need surgery to remove a piece of diseased bowel or drain an abscess that has developed. How do you know when you need surgery?

- You are not responding to therapy with medications, and you are getting sicker.
- You've developed a narrowing of the bowel, perhaps from a buildup of scar tissue on the bowel wall, that's obstructing the flow of digested food.
- You have adhesions—scar tissue where damaged bowel is incorrectly healing together—that are pulling or kinking the bowel and causing obstruction.
- The products of inflammation are obstructing your bowel.
- Inflammation has eaten through the bowel wall and caused perforation and abscess.
- You have a fistula that won't heal on its own.
- You have dysplasia or cancer.
- You have a hemorrhage, which requires emergency repair, fortunately a very rare occurrence these days.

Resection

A resection is the process of removing a portion of the small and/or large intestine. It is a generic term that surgeons use to describe what they do.

Fixing Perforation or Abscess

Because Crohn's involves inflammation of all the layers of the bowel, when damage spans the entire bowel wall, you can "spring a leak." This is known as a perforation, which is a hole or tear. Perforations lead to abscesses, because stool and bacteria leak out of the bowel to form the abscess. As you might guess, this causes infection.

Symptoms of a perforation depend on how big the hole is. Sudden abdominal pain, fever, nausea, and vomiting are all common symptoms of a perforation. An abscess can stay hidden for a while, depending on where it develops. The abdominal cavity can accommodate a growing abscess for a few days before symptoms may come to your attention. Low-grade fevers, vague pain, or even the inability to straighten out the leg without pain are all symptoms of an abscess. If the abscess is positioned near the abdominal muscles that help keep the body upright or the leg straight, these can be the only symptoms. Sometimes, abscesses are only found when a CT scan is done.

In Crohn's, if the hole is small enough, you can sometimes use medicine to patch it. Antibiotics to fight the infection and biologics and immunosuppressants to stop the inflammation working together can promote healing. As you do with a leaky pipe in the basement, at first you patch it or put duct tape over the leak, but when the water comes out around the patch job, you usually replace that piece of leaky pipe. Sometimes with a perforation, it is best to just cut that part of the bowel out and sew the healthy tissue together.

Repairing Anal Fistulas

Another problem that can occur in Crohn's disease is a fistula around the anal area. Because of the inflammation that burrows through all layers of the bowel and rectal wall, breakdown around the anal canal can occur. A fistula can start as some pain around the anal canal, a sensation of pressure, and then even a feeling of fluid draining, which can be blood, stool, or pus. Sitting in a warm bath can help relieve the pressure and allow the area to drain if small enough.

Sometimes, however, pus can build up in the area, and it needs to be drained by a surgeon. In this instance, the surgeon may not only drain the area but put in a temporary drain to help evacuate all the pus. He or she may also place a seton in the fistula tract itself to allow it to freely drain so that an abscess cannot form. Setons are simply rubber bands that are sewn into place as a temporary measure while medical therapy helps to heal the inflammation around that area and close the fistula tract. They are removed once the area is no longer inflamed. Sometimes setons are adjusted, particularly for large fistula tracts that are taking longer to heal. A surgeon will adjust the seton so that it is not as loose as the fistula tract gets smaller and smaller before eventual removal. This process does not hurt, as the band is simply running through the area, and unless the tract completely closes, the healing tissue does not adhere to it. Complete closure is rare in the time frame in which most people have a seton in place. Setons can stay in place for long periods (months to years) if a fistula tract is proving to be quite resistant to closing. Some people have a seton in for years. Because it prevents abscesses from recurring, it's not removed until the fistula is healed enough to no longer be at risk for abscess formation. A seton can be removed in the office; it is pulled out just like stitches would be after a common surgery.

Hemorrhoids: Consider Surgery Last

Large hemorrhoids or "skin tags" around the anal canal are a common complaint in those with Crohn's disease. Skin tags usually are not felt unless they are swollen, and usually it takes an experienced pair of eyes to determine whether these are simply skin tags or are hemorrhoids. Skin tags are benign extra growths of anal tissue, whereas hemorrhoids are swollen blood vessels of the anal canal. Some people have both, which makes the situation more confusing.

External hemorrhoids are found around the outside of the anal canal and can be mistaken for skin tags. Internal hemorrhoids are not visible with the naked eye and aren't felt on physical exam unless very swollen. Either kind of hemorrhoid can be particularly bothersome when you're dealing with diarrhea because the irritation of stool passage and the wiping can cause pain, swelling, and bleeding.

Skin tags are not regular hemorrhoids and are considered one of the symptoms of Crohn's. Treatment includes topical creams for discomfort, control of diarrhea, and treatment of the underlying Crohn's disease. When we remove hemorrhoids in people with Crohn's disease, there is a higher rate of complications like scarring, bleeding, and infection so this surgery is usually not recommended. It's important to discuss your concerns with your gastroenterology health care provider. If you are contemplating hemorrhoid surgery, you must see an experienced colorectal surgeon who understands Crohn's disease.

Postoperative Complications

All surgery carries with it some risk. Some are related to undergoing surgery in general, whereas others are related to having surgery on the bowels specifically.

Ileus

This is the term used when the bowel remains "asleep" after anesthesia and does not regain function quickly. We do not know why some people take longer for their bowels to wake up and start moving. Eventually the bowel does wake up, but it can take close to 30 days for this to occur. Normally, the bowels wake up within 3 to 5 days.

There are a few things that can increase your risk for ileus: if your surgery is very involved or complicated and requires a lot of manipulation of the bowel, if it takes a long time to complete, if you were taking narcotics before surgery that slowed down the bowels before the surgery, if you are taking a large amount of narcotics after surgery for pain control, or if you are in poor general health. Maneuvers that are thought to help get the bowels moving again include walking, deep breathing, sucking on hard candy, and for some, chewing gum.

Thrombosis or Blood Clots

Manipulation of the bowel, remaining immobile after surgery, and intravenous catheters lead to blood pooling in the veins and can cause clots. Clots in the large veins of the abdomen can cause pain and loss of blood flow from the intestines. This can interfere with the healing of the connections that were created during surgery. Clots in the legs can cause pain, swelling, and redness of the leg. These clots can migrate from the legs through the blood vessels to the lungs, which is life threatening. People with IBD are at greater risk for blood clot formation than the rest of the population, especially if you have very active disease. It is still unclear why this occurs, but it is an important problem that we need to monitor for after an operation.

To avoid ileus and thrombosis, it's important for you to get up and get moving as quickly as you can after surgery to help the bowels wake up and keep your blood flowing. Even just sitting up and dangling your legs at the side of the bed or getting up to sit in a chair are important steps to postoperative recovery. Taking slow, deep breaths to fill the lungs with air is also important.

Bowel Obstruction from Adhesions

Soon after abdominal surgery, scar tissue starts to form. Sometimes, scar tissue grows so that it connects one place on the bowel with another loop of bowel or the abdominal wall. Often, an adhesion causes no problems; but sometimes, the bowel will kink on that band of scar tissue, which creates an obstruction. This is not due to Crohn's, but instead is a mechanical problem. This does not happen more often in people with Crohn's disease and is part of the natural process of healing. An obstruction will cause nausea, vomiting, and abdominal pain and may seem just like a flare of disease, except that you will also cease to pass any stool or gas. We usually treat obstructions with bowel rest and possibly a tube into the stomach to decompress the trapped fluid, but sometimes, if the obstruction does not undo itself, surgery is required to unkink the bowel and cut away the scar tissue that has caused the kinking.

Other Surgical Complications

Wound infection. If you are using steroids and need to have surgery, your risk for poor wound healing and infection increases, just like people with diabetes. Steroids cause thinning of the skin and blood vessels, which makes them more sensitive to manipulation and damage even with minimal manipulation.

Abscess. An abscess is a collection of fluid and cells that are basically the products of the immune response that are created to fight infection. Abscesses occur due to a wound infection or a new infection at the site of surgical connection of the bowels. We use antibiotics to control the infection and, depending on the size and location, the area may need to be drained with a drain placed using a CT scan for guidance or by a surgeon.

Anastomotic leaking. There are several reasons why the site of the reconnection of the bowels may come apart. These include too much tension on the connection, poor healing from steroids, infection, or residual active disease. When this happens, you'll have pain and fever and possibly an abscess will form; this requires another operation.

Anastomotic ischemia. This is poor blood flow to the site of the bowel surgery. If the reconnection between two pieces of bowel is pulled too tight, the area doesn't receive enough blood flow, which causes damage and bleeding. When there is inadequate blood flow to the area, it is like having a heart attack; the cells start to die, and the heart cannot pump blood. This is different from the ulceration in active Crohn's disease.

Acute narcotic withdrawal. If you were taking large doses of narcotics before the surgery, you may not receive equivalent amounts following surgery and experience worsening pain, nausea, vomiting, and even personality changes and hallucinations from narcotic withdrawal. Minimizing the amount of narcotics before the surgery and being honest about the amount you take when you are discussing surgery will help you avoid such a complication.

Acute steroid withdrawal. If you were taking high doses of steroids before surgery, you may suffer withdrawal if postoperatively you do not receive the same amounts intravenously while recovering. Sleep and personality changes and electrolyte imbalances can occur in this situation. Fortunately, surgeons are specially trained to follow protocols for steroid dosing during and after surgeries.

Diarrhea. This can happen from the loss of absorptive surface when there has been bowel removal or because a blockage was corrected. Depending on the cause, intervention is necessary, but sometimes it resolves on its own within a few days.

Long-Term Complications of Small Intestine Surgery

When you need to have some or most of your small intestine removed, predictable problems occur. First, you can develop bile salt diarrhea. Bile, which is released by the liver to help you digest fat, is normally absorbed in the small intestine. Normally it gets removed from digested food before it reaches the colon. When too much of the small intestine is gone, there is a higher chance of some bile getting into the colon. Bile irritates the lining of the colon, which responds by producing a watery diarrhea. Medications like cholestyramine can help (see Chapter 6) because they bind bile so that it does not reach the colon.

Second, you can suffer nutritional losses. The only place in the body that can absorb vitamin B_{12} from food is the terminal ileum. B_{12} is needed for almost every function of the body. In Crohn's disease, when the terminal ileum is inflamed or has been removed, it can no longer absorb vitamin B_{12} from the diet, so it's important to get it from shots every 1 to 3 months or with a special nasal spray. Folate is another nutrient that can become depleted from surgery, so make sure that your levels are monitored after surgery to check for deficiencies. There is more about nutrition in Chapter 10.

Finally, *short bowel syndrome* is a special situation that occurs in a small number of people with Crohn's disease. Normally, we have about 300 centimeters of small intestine. When you only have 100 centimeters or less left, you usually are not able to absorb all the water and nutrients you need to survive. The risk for dehydration and complications from vitamin deficiencies is high, and monitoring by a nutrition specialist is vital. Typically, you'll need intravenous support with total parenteral nutrition (TPN). How do you know if you have short bowel syndrome? An X-ray can measure the approximate length of your small intestine. There are no special symptoms associated with a short bowel, because the diarrhea and vitamin deficiencies associated with short bowel syndrome can also happen for other reasons.

Stoma

No one wants a stoma but you should understand about them. There are several different kinds. The most common is an ileostomy, which is an opening from the ileum to the abdominal wall. Output from this is semiliquid waste, as well as gas, and because it does not interact with any bacteria, it has much less odor than regular stool. You need to empty the bag frequently because the liquid fills it multiple times a day. It's easy to become dehydrated; you might not realize that you have to replace the fluid that comes out of the stoma each day.

FIGURE 9. Typical Ileostomy

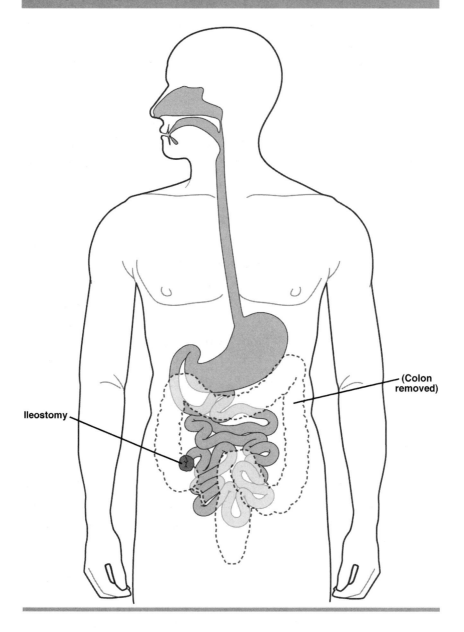

Ileostomy

(Colon removed)

A colostomy, which most people commonly call any form of stoma with a bag, comes off the colon. We use a colostomy when someone with Crohn's disease has a damaged portion of the colon that cannot be sewn back together. In this case, the waste is stool, which may have odor, but you don't have to empty the bag as frequently. This kind of surgery is less common in IBD and more common due to other conditions that occur in older patients, such as colon cancer and diverticulitis. The third kind of pouch is a jejunostomy, which originates from the central portion of the small intestine. This fluid contains a lot of electrolytes, and management of this stoma is the most difficult. This kind of stoma is fortunately very uncommon, but occurs when so much of the ileum is diseased that it has to be bypassed.

If you need a stoma, you'll get to know a stoma/wound care nurse, who is a specialty nurse trained in the care and education of patients with stomas—of all kinds. These nurses are usually affiliated with a hospital but some of the busier surgeons may have one in their practice. If you have the opportunity, before having any surgery where you might possibly end up with an ostomy, be sure to meet with a stoma nurse to be evaluated for the best place to put the stoma. The nurse will mark this site so that the surgeon knows exactly where the best fit will be. Generally, this is under the belt line so that clothes or a belt won't rub on the stoma and cause trauma. Even in emergency situations, there is time for a stoma nurse to mark your abdomen for a reasonable site for a stoma. Make sure you ask about seeing the nurse before your surgery.

Following surgery, the stoma nurse will help you learn how to care for your stoma. You need follow-up visits to make sure the appliance that holds the bag in place has a good fit and that your skin underneath the adhesive is not damaged. When the adhesive seal or appliance is loose, waste material can leak and further damage the skin. When individuals gain or lose a significant amount of weight, the stoma and its outer appliance may change shape or lose its original fitting and should be re-evaluated.

There is another surgical procedure that is done by only a few surgeons around the country where a "continent ostomy" is created. This is also made from the small intestine, but the pouch is not attached to the anal canal; instead, it exits the body on the anterior abdominal wall in the right lower quadrant. There is an external "nipple" that is catheterized on a regular basis throughout the day to drain out the contents of the pouch. You don't wear an external bag. This surgery is highly specialized and can be associated with a lot of complications and so it is not the preferred surgical choice for anyone needing the entire colon removed.

Other Surgeries

Considering the increasing rate of obesity in the United States, there is the possibility that you may have IBD and also be a candidate for obesity surgery. If you have ulcerative colitis, bypass surgery is acceptable, but you need to know that if you have a flare and develop diarrhea, your risk of dehydration is greater. If you have Crohn's disease, neither bypass or stomach stapling surgery is a good idea. Diarrhea can develop because the normal, healthy tissue has been bypassed, and it is much easier for you to become malnourished. Therefore, if you need surgical weight loss, the lap band is much more appropriate, because it is reversible.

For other types of surgeries that you might need to plan for, such as joint repair, hysterectomy, or gallbladder removal, talk to your health care provider about which medications you may have to stop before the surgery and when you can start taking them again. If you are on steroids, make sure your surgeon knows this, as you may need extra steroids during the operation.

To sum up, surgery can offer you a way to improve your health, but you need to have it in the right circumstances, by the right surgeon. If you are really ill and have had troubles with medical therapy, you are more likely to suffer complications from surgery as well. Also, bear in mind that surgery is usually not reversible. Because of this, if you are able, discuss your options in detail before you make this decision. Your surgeon should be working closely with your other health care providers to maximize your health outcomes.

10

The Food Fight: What Can I Eat?

Coauthored by Susan Hopson, RD

Among the many wide-ranging challenges of having inflammatory bowel disease (IBD), the one most likely to cause you frustration is figuring out how and what to eat. If this area of IBD self-management has been the hardest for you, that is more often the case than not. More time is spent discussing diet with patients than any other topic.

Before your symptoms of IBD began, it was reasonable for you to assume that the dietary guidelines of the major health organizations would successfully guide your body toward good health, especially in your digestive tract. Eating may have been a wonderful source of pleasure for you. But living with IBD presents you with a range of new challenges that require new approaches to eating. The modified guidelines will, however, help you to get all the nutrition your body needs and, at the same time, help you make some peace with food.

We all know what it's like to eat things that don't agree with us, so we avoid them. You might reasonably conclude that, when your GI tract is hurting from an IBD flare, choosing different foods would be the key to making it better. While that is partly true, life with IBD isn't that simple. Let's take a look at whether you can use what you eat to treat your IBD.

Your Nutritional Challenge

If you broke your leg, you could find a way to get around without using that leg until it healed. However, if you had a heart attack, you would have to take special steps to repair your heart and to keep from having another attack, all the while depending on your heart to continue beating. Similarly, with IBD, your primary organ for digesting and absorbing food is damaged. It functions, but it doesn't function very well at times. However, you depend on your gut to provide your body with the nutrients you need to survive.

There are several reasons why your body may not receive all the nutrition it needs. For example, during a flare a portion of your gut's lining is inflamed, which may reduce its ability to adequately absorb nutrients. At the same time, because of the inflammation, your need for nutrients becomes greater. This is because the flare increases loss of gut tissue, which needs to be replaced. In addition to needing nutrients for the new tissue, the inflammation raises your metabolic rate, which means you are burning calories faster than when you are not sick. Your metabolism is the rate at which your body "engine" runs. Energy from food is converted into a form of energy that your body can use to perform all its many functions. One of these is tissue repair.

In addition, your gut may have narrowed areas that make it difficult for food to pass through. This results in cramping and pain. Some sections may have ceased to function at all, or portions may have been surgically removed. Both can result in poor absorption of water and bile salts, which leads to diarrhea. You may be avoiding certain nutritious foods because they are associated with past unpleasant or embarrassing episodes when you couldn't get to a bathroom in time.

Nutrition 101: What Every Body Needs

Humans need six essential nutrients to survive: carbohydrates, protein, fat, vitamins, minerals, and water. The fact that our bodies cannot make any of these is the reason they are called "essential." We need to obtain these nutrients from the environment.

Carbohydrates, protein, and fat, known in the nutrition world as macronutrients, provide the calories that we use for our energy and are needed in quantities large enough to be measured in grams or ounces. Vitamins and minerals are necessary only in very small amounts, hundredths or even millionths of a gram, and so are called *micronutrients*. They contain no calories. Finally, we need water, or liquids that contain water, most of all. It's a fact that staying adequately hydrated is more important for life than keeping fed.

You may associate "carbs" with bread and potatoes, protein with meat, and fat with oil or grease. Although these associations are not incorrect, they are incomplete. Most foods are combinations of carbohydrates, protein, and fat, and in addition, contain various combinations of vitamins, minerals, and water.

Carbohydrates

In this book, the term *carbohydrate* refers to the chemical compound, or nutrient, in foods, not the more common usage that denotes carbohydrate-containing foods such as potatoes, bread, and rice. Generally speaking, carbohydrates are sugars and starches; one type of starch is fiber. They provide mostly energy (calories) and are found in varying quantities in anything made with grains, fruit, milk, vegetables, and nuts. We get very few calories from fiber because it's not absorbed. However, fiber plays a role in IBD management that it is important to understand, so it is addressed beginning on page 150. There are no carbohydrates in meat or fat unless they added during food preparation, which is why the famous "low-carb diets" rely on a heavy intake of meat and fat. Most foods that are categorized as carbohydrates contain vitamins and a few minerals. Most nutrition experts say that a healthy, well-balanced diet has between half and three quarters of its foods as carbohydrates, although this really varies by individual needs.

Proteins

Proteins are found mainly in meat (including fish and poultry), eggs, milk and milk products, beans, and nuts. In addition, most starches and vegetables have a few grams of protein. Our bodies require a lot of protein, somewhere in the range of 12% to 30% of our daily intake of food. Protein provides the structural components of our bodies. Proteins in the form of enzymes and hormones and in genetic information (DNA, RNA) carry information throughout our bodies. Among other things, proteins tell our cells and organs how to assemble and disassemble themselves and what actions they should perform. Proteins do a lot! They come in many shapes and take on many different roles.

Fat

Fat is simpler in both shape and function than protein. This nutrient includes solid fats, oils, and waxes, the first two being the fats we are most likely to eat. Fats store energy in a very concentrated form for later use. Consider that a gram of fat contains more than twice as many calories as a gram of carbohydrate or protein. In the popular media, fats have a bad reputation because of their high calorie levels, but they play an important role in our health and deserve more respect. A healthy diet has 20% to 35% of calories as fats.

Like proteins, fats come in different forms: saturated, monounsaturated, and polyunsaturated. A diet high in saturated fat is associated with heart disease and obesity. The healthier oils—the unsaturated types—can help turn inflammation on and off (remember that inflammation is an important way to maintain overall health), keep cholesterol levels under control, allow the brain to develop normal connections (a vital function in babies and young children), and maintain those connections, especially as we age. Fats also deliver to our tissues a few vitamins that cannot be broken down and carried in water. Finally, they provide us with insulation to keep us warm and help cushion our organs in case of blows and jostling.

Polyunsaturated fats include the omega-3 and omega-6 fatty acids that you may have heard about. Eicosapentaenoic acid (EPA) and docosahexaenoic acid (DHA) are both omega-3 fatty acids found in fish oil that may be beneficial to those with IBD. Omega-3 fatty acids have anti-inflammatory properties and may decrease both active inflammation and the rate of relapse in those with Crohn's disease who are in remission (see Chapter 6).[177–185] Trials performed in Europe showed that omega-3 supplements could treat the active symptoms of Crohn's. Unfortunately, the formulation of fish oil used in those trials is not available in the U.S. and is equivalent to eating 2 to 3 pounds of fish per day. Two other studies using omega-3 supplements after surgery to maintain inflammation remission did not show any benefit over placebo. So, it remains unclear how we should use omega-3 in the treatment of Crohn's disease, especially when and at what dose. Supplementing your diet with omega-3 provides an anti-inflammatory action, which is healthy. The recommended daily dose depends on the formulation, but taking it appears at least safe and perhaps of overall benefit. It is thought that following a Mediterranean-style diet, including fish and olive oil, is beneficial for patients with IBD. On the other hand, it's better to avoid omega-6 fatty acids (safflower oil, corn oil, walnuts), as they have properties that promote inflammation.

Vitamins

Our good health and survival depends on getting from our food the 13 essential vitamins that our bodies are unable to make. These vitamins have multiple functions and allow a variety of reactions to occur within our tissues, whether breaking things down for use or disposal or building things up to become part of our bodies or something else we can use. The B vitamins and vitamin C are water soluble and are absorbed and carried with water in our blood. Vitamins A, D, E, and K must be present in the fat in our food in order to be absorbed, and then are carried, attached to fat molecules, in our blood to reach the cells that need them.

Minerals

Minerals perform a surprising number of roles. Here is just a partial sample. Calcium is incorporated into our bones, but among other things, it also helps blood to clot and our heart to beat. Iron combines with oxygen and carries it in our blood to our tissues, where the oxygen is released. Sodium and potassium control the amount and location of water in our bodies. Potassium helps our muscles contract. Copper is found in enzymes that drive certain vital reactions—and that can't occur if we don't have enough copper. Copper is also a component of hormones and helps to make red blood cells. Except for a few, like calcium and magnesium, most minerals are needed in very small quantities, but needed they are. It pays to take them seriously. Most people with IBD won't have problems getting the minerals needed in small quantities, but everyone should consume 1,200 mg of calcium per day with at least 800 International Units (IUs) of vitamin D per day.

Your Individual Nutrition Needs

A great deal of research over the last 100 years has enabled the major health organizations to reach fairly close agreement about how much carbohydrate, protein, and fat the average human needs in order to remain healthy. But the fact is that individuals vary. Your genetic makeup and your environment work together to determine how much of a particular vitamin or mineral—or even fats, carbohydrates, and protein—your body needs at any particular time. For example, because of your IBD, you need more protein when you are having or recovering from a bout of inflammation. That's because your body uses protein to repair itself. Also, you need more vitamin C when you are under stress or have wounds that must heal.

Because IBD is a nutritionally demanding condition, it is a good idea to take a multivitamin each day unless your health care provider tells you otherwise. There are some multivitamins that are specifically formulated for patients with IBD (Forvia) as they contain more vitamin B_{12}, iron, and folic acid than others. But unless you notice a difference or have a specific deficiency that needs treating, you do not need special vitamins, which cost more. You can find a complete multivitamin at the store that you find palatable. For those who do need extra folic acid and iron, consider a prenatal vitamin, which works even if you are not contemplating pregnancy or are male. Some people, particularly postmenopausal women or people who are lactose intolerant, need to take additional calcium and vitamin D.

IBD-Required Modifications

When your disease is active, you might be modifying your diet, and if it makes you feel better, you undoubtedly will not mind doing that. However, even after the inflammatory stage is over and you are feeling better again, you may find that certain foods continue to irritate your gut and, in the case of "trigger" foods, may even cause a flare. You will want to continue to avoid those foods all or most of the time.

There are foods that need to be off limits at certain times but eaten as much as you can tolerate the rest of the time. Fiber is the most obvious: during a flare, you want to avoid it, but once you are healed, fiber is part of a healthy diet.[234] You may also need to avoid certain foods during a flare that ordinarily would not bother you, such as dairy, some herbs and spices, even hot or cold foods. You may have to eat smaller, more frequent meals so as not to distend your bowel with bulk and gas.

Although red meat is particularly high in fat, it is an excellent source of protein and iron. Your body requires protein to help heal the damage to your bowel caused by inflammation. The important thing to remember about red meat is that the body can only digest about 6 ounces at any given meal. When the smallest steak at a restaurant is 9 ounces, this might seem like a small portion. But eat too much and you may flood your bowel with hard-to-digest fat, which leads to bloating, pain, and diarrhea. Essentially, a typical large hamburger served at a fast-food restaurant is as much red meat as you should try to ingest at a meal.

In addition, there may be foods to which you alone are sensitive, that make you uncomfortable, or just seem to make you feel worse all over. After a flare and once your symptoms have resolved, you can often enjoy them again. It is particularly important to increase your intake of fiber if at all possible; most of us don't meet the nutritional guidelines for fiber.

Your diet will probably face more modifications if you have Crohn's disease than if you have ulcerative colitis. This is because the tissue damage from Crohn's disease usually occurs in those areas of the small intestine most involved in nutrient absorption, thus preventing uptake of the nutrients needed for repair. Finally, drug treatments for Crohn's disease cause loss of nutrients and, at the same time, increase your need for protein.

Learn to let experience be your guide. There is much you can do to help keep your IBD under control by being observant of trends and connections. How good are you at paying attention to the signals that your body provides about when you feel better or worse, or when you have more energy or less, or how often you are getting ill? These things are not necessarily due to nutrition, but they may be. It is a good idea to learn to notice.

Although some restrictions—fiber, for example—are common to nearly everyone with IBD, it helps to keep a food diary until you learn how you, individually, respond to different foods (Figure 10). Your diary is where you keep track of the kinds of food you eat, when you ate them, and approximately how much. Then, when symptoms occur, write down the time and a description of how you feel. Over time, you will probably see trends, that certain foods and certain symptoms occur together, one following the other. Having this information will make it much easier to stay away from those foods and feel better. This is a very good tool to learn effective IBD self-management.

Fiber and Residue

Almost all of the nutrients in the food we consume are extracted from the food while in the small intestine. There, the nutrients pass into our bloodstream for delivery to the cells throughout our bodies. The

FIGURE 10. Sample Food Diary		
Time	**Food/Amount**	**Symptom**
8:00 a.m.	black coffee, 1 cup orange juice oatmeal with milk	
10:30	muffin	
11:30		diarrhea, cramps
1:00 p.m.	fruit smoothie	
4:00		*bad* diarrhea
6:00	green beans rice BBQ pork chop tossed salad	
8:00		pain, cramping
10:00	oatmeal cookie	
3:00 a.m.		explosive bm, mucus, cramps

remainder of the food, nearly all plant material, continues on through the GI tract. This plant material is what we refer to as fiber and what your grandparents probably called *roughage*. It is primarily the structural parts of plants like the cell walls, which are mostly indigestible carbohydrates and a little lignin. Although starches are also carbohydrates, they are digestible and therefore are not considered to be fiber.

"Residue" is another term you may occasionally encounter. It includes not only fiber, but all the contents that remain in the large intestine: other undigested food, bacteria, intestinal secretions, and intestinal cells that have sloughed off as they are replaced by new cells. Sometimes a low-fiber diet is called a low-residue diet because residue can act as stool-bulking agent, but this use can be confusing. Think of residue like the soap residue on the shower tile; this residue in your intestines can build up and cause bloating and discomfort—and potentially a blockage if there is a stricture present.

Solubility and Insolubility

Fiber is divided into two types, soluble and insoluble. Simply put, fiber is one type or the other depending on whether it will dissolve in water. That is a bit of an oversimplification, but it is accurate enough for a broad understanding of how each kind of fiber is treated and used by your body. The two fibers act somewhat differently in our bodies and perform different functions, each important to bowel health.

Fiber passes through the esophagus, stomach, and small intestine unaffected by our digestive enzymes. Insoluble fiber is, however, broken into smaller and smaller pieces by chewing, stomach acid, and the rough-and-tumble churning of our intestinal contractions. Soluble fiber dissolves in the water in the gut. Although fiber is not digested in the small intestine, it still performs useful functions in the upper digestive tract, for example, slowing down stomach emptying and lengthening the time it takes for the sugar in a meal to be absorbed. Generally, these actions have a beneficial effect on how we feel.

Fiber that dissolves in water produces a smooth, almost slimy slurry that moves slowly through the gut. If you can imagine the texture of a finely ground oatmeal after it has been cooked in water and allowed to cool for awhile, you get the idea. Insoluble fiber, on the other hand, keeps its rough texture and is anything but smooth and slippery. It moves much more quickly through the intestine than does soluble fiber, and as it travels, it scrapes off the old cells that line the intestine so they can be replaced by new ones.

When it reaches the large intestine, some of the fiber is digested after all—not by our digestive enzymes, but by "good" bacteria that reside there in a mutually beneficial relationship with us. We provide the bacteria with food in the form of soluble fiber, and they, in turn, convert the fiber into short-chain fatty acids (SCFA) that the cells in our colons use for their energy. Our colons must have SCFAs to survive and stay healthy. However, the bacterial digestion of fiber also produces water and gas. This is one of the reasons why we feel unusually bloated and gassy after eating a high-fiber meal, especially if we are not accustomed to it.

Both types of fiber absorb several times more water than their own volume, which makes the stool bulkier, softer, and easier to pass. But, because of their bulk, fiber and residue stretch (distend) your bowel, which can be uncomfortable when it is inflamed and sensitive. Add this to the products of bacterial digestion, and you can understand why you want to avoid fiber during a flare, when just the contractile action that moves the fecal mass through the intestine can hurt. Some of the harsher fibers also cause a mild scraping of the tissues, something you wouldn't notice if the tissues were intact and healthy but which can cause pain when they are not.

Fiber is good for you and, especially for its role as the producer of SCFAs, is a necessary component of a healthy diet.[235] It is one of those foods that your body needs for long-term gut health but, at certain times, you must avoid in order to give your inflamed gut a rest. As you can see, it pays to be fiber "savvy"!

Fiber Guidelines

The American Dietetic Association recommends that adults consume a minimum of 25 to 35 grams of fiber each day and that children take in the number of grams of fiber each day equal to their age plus 5. Because food labels give the amount of fiber per serving, it's easy to develop a sense of how much fiber you eat from packaged foods.

You will probably be able to eat the recommended amount of fiber when your IBD is inactive and your bowel is not inflamed. But some people with IBD find that eating fiber is a problem regardless of disease activity. If you are just learning how to deal with IBD, use a food diary to keep track of your fiber intake. You want to make sure that you are getting a healthy amount but also watch for trends in the activity of your disease. Try not to let yourself feel that fiber is "the enemy." Fiber does much to keep your gut cells healthy and to prevent relapses, provided you consume it when your gut is able to deal with it.

Adding Fiber In

If you are recovering from an inflammatory episode and your doctor has instructed you to increase your fiber intake, there are two "rules of thumb" to remember. The first is to increase your intake *very slowly,* only a few grams more each week than the week before. For example, you might try ¼ cup of oatmeal for soluble fiber and a ¼ piece of whole wheat toast for insoluble fiber. Skip a day and do it again. Then, increase it to every day. After a week, double the amount of oatmeal and add a few small pieces of canned fruit or a ½ cup of a soft, thin-skinned vegetable that you've been missing. Continue in this way until you have reached the amount your health care provider recommends.

The second rule is to drink lots of fluid, enough to keep your urine a very pale yellow. If it is bright yellow, you are not getting enough water. Fiber absorbs water, which keeps it soft and easy to pass. If there is not enough water available for it to absorb, severe, uncomfortable constipation can result.

If you have a lot of flares, fiber is obviously an important thing for you to manage well. Consider investing in one of the many books available that list foods and their fiber contents. Some are small enough to fit into a pocket or purse. They can be quite handy when you are unsure which choices to make. If you need more fiber but are unsure what you can eat to get it, consider one of many fiber supplements. They come in the form of tablets, capsules, granules, and cereals. Each is clearly labeled as to the amount of each kind of fiber it provides.

Lactose Intolerance

Lactose is a sugar that is a natural component of milk. If you have Crohn's disease, your doctor may have told you to avoid lactose or you may have already figured out for yourself that milk or milk products cause you problems. Lactose intolerance is the inability to digest lactose. For many adults and almost all children, lactose is digested in the small intestine and broken down by an enzyme produced there called lactase. If your small intestine is inflamed or damaged, you are less likely to have enough lactase to digest milk. If you have ulcerative colitis, it is less likely that you would be lactose intolerant because the inflammation is in your colon rather than small intestine. There is a great deal of variation between people, however, in their sensitivity to lactose. Sometimes the condition is only temporary, and sometimes it is permanent. Also, individuals may tolerate varying amounts of milk at different times.

If you are lactose intolerant and drink milk or eat food with milk in it, it will probably give you some, or all, of the following symptoms: gas, bloating, loose and urgent bowel movements, mucus in your stool, cramping, and pain. In addition to matching lactose exposure to your symptoms, hydrogen breath testing is a way to diagnose lactose intolerance. Lactose that you were unable to digest is digested by bacteria in your colon that create byproducts, one of which is hydrogen. The extra hydrogen is carried in the bloodstream to the lungs and shows up at abnormally high levels in your breath.

Lactose intolerance does not only affect people with IBD. In fact, approximately 70% to 90% of the world's population is lactose intolerant as adults! The ability to digest milk is most important to babies, and babies the world over have no problem doing so. After infancy, however, most cultures of the world do not drink much milk, and the enzyme lactase is no longer needed and so is no longer produced. In general, our bodies don't waste energy and resources producing things we don't need. A tolerance for lactose is actually the "abnormal" condition. Interestingly, the highest percentages of adults in any country (97%) that can tolerate milk are found in Sweden and Denmark. Scientists propose that, in northern latitudes, this may be to their advantage. They experience the lowest levels of the sunlight required for their skin to produce vitamin D, which is needed for calcium absorption, so calcium levels are lowered. Lactose enhances calcium absorption, which is likely the reason why lactose tolerance was retained in the genes of the Northern Europeans. The populations of South America, Africa, Asia, and Mediterranean regions, all areas of abundant sunlight, as well as those who have emigrated from these areas to North America and Europe, rarely tolerate milk and utilize cuisines that depend on other sources for protein, calcium, and vitamin D.

If you are lactose intolerant and your disease is active, it's important to stop drinking milk or eating products with any milk in them altogether. This means totally avoiding regular or flavored milks, evaporated or condensed milk, ice cream or frozen yogurt, buttermilk, cream soups, cheese and perhaps butter, and milk-based pudding. These sources will be fairly obvious to you and not too difficult to avoid. However, there are less obvious sources that include casein (the solid part of milk), whey (the liquid part of milk), and milk solids, so be sure to check the list of ingredients on food labels. Finally, you need to be aware of the truly sneaky sources of milk: drugs and supplements that use lactose as a filler. Again, read the labels and, if unsure, ask your pharmacist.

Once the inflammation in your gut has settled down and you are again able to include more options in your list of tolerable foods, it may be safe for you to try reintroducing milk into your diet. Most people with lactose intolerance can eventually tolerate somewhere between ½ and 1 cup of milk in a day without unpleasant symptoms. Do not expect or try to do this immediately, however.

Lactaid is a brand of milk available in most grocery stores. It has lactose-digesting enzymes added to it, which makes it acceptable in small quantities, such as added to coffee, poured on cereal, or added to soups. Look for it in the cooler section near the other kinds of milk.

There are also products in the form of lactase drops that you can add to regular milk 24 hours before drinking it. They break down some, but not all, of the lactose. Some people have been successful at breaking down even more of the lactase by heating the milk and doubling the usual dose of drops, then allowing it to sit overnight in the refrigerator. This may be worth a try if you really enjoy having a glass of milk.

Some yogurt contains bacteria that break down lactose. Try a few spoonfuls, and see what happens. If you have no symptoms in the next two days, try again with a little more. Eventually you may be able to tolerate as much as a small carton without symptoms.

Lactase pills are available over the counter at most pharmacies and in many grocery stores. With these, you chew two or three pills immediately before eating or drinking foods containing milk. Timing is the key to using these pills. If you take them too soon, your stomach will break down the enzymes (your stomach considers them just another protein to digest), rendering them ineffective. It is wise to carry some with you in case you find yourself faced with more milk than you think you can handle. They don't break down all the lactose present, but they help. This may allow you to eat foods in which lactose is listed as an ingredient—certain breads, sherbets, or restaurant dishes with cheese, for example.

Finally, there are other kinds of "milk" besides cow's milk that contain no lactose. Soy, rice, and almond milks can be found in most large supermarkets. They are perfectly okay for you to use, at least in terms of lactose.

It will be a matter of trial and error but, with patience and careful record keeping, you may find that living with lactose intolerance is not difficult. After all, you have 70% of the world's population to keep you company!

Calcium: A Special Problem

The absorptive lining of your small intestine—the villi—may be so damaged during the active phase of the disease that it may not function much at all. So it is easy for you to become deficient in a number of nutrients. Calcium poses a special problem. There are other vitamins and minerals present in milk that we need to consume, but these are found abundantly in other foods. However, our bodies need a lot of calcium, and milk is the most concentrated food source of that mineral.

Even when you are able to consume milk again, you may find you don't want to. After a few bouts of gas, cramps, flatulence, and urgent, mucus-filled stools, you can easily begin to associate milk with unpleasantness and lose the desire to drink it. As a consequence, your calcium intake becomes lower still.

The drugs used to suppress the inflammation in the GI tract, such as steroids, methotrexate, and cyclosporine, cause calcium to be lost from bones, making you especially prone to osteopenia or even osteoporosis. Between malabsorption, reduced intake, and calcium loss from bones, calcium deficiency can be severe. Calcium fuels many processes in your body in addition to keeping your bones strong, so it's vital to take this seriously and increase your intake of other food sources of calcium.

Also, because vitamin D helps calcium to be deposited in bone, it pays to increase that as well. Under ideal conditions, people manufacture vitamin D in their skin when it is exposed to sunlight. If you live in a southern sunny climate, you are less likely to be deficient in this vitamin, but people vary in the amount of vitamin D they are able to produce from this source. Although there are some good food sources that can be utilized, it is generally recommended that you take oral supplements of both calcium and vitamin D. The current recommendation for calcium is 1,200 mg per day for adults and the new, updated recommendation for vitamin D is 1,000 IUs a day—a big increase over the 200 IUs we used to think we needed. However, the truth is that your body absorbs vitamins and minerals more easily from food, so the more you can get in that way, the better.

Here are some nondairy sources of calcium:

- Eggs
- Canned salmon with bones. Eat the bones! The canning processes makes them soft and easily chewed. If the somewhat gritty nature of the bones bothers you, or if you must avoid anything potentially abrasive, mash them with a spoon or even put them through a blender. This is tedious, but will provide you with a lot of calcium. Eventually, ease of preparation will probably win out over distaste, and you will probably get used to eating the bones as they are.
- Soy from calcium-enriched soy milk, regular and firm tofu, soy "cheeses"
- Leafy greens like spinach and collards and vegetables like kale and broccoli. You may not always be able to tolerate the fiber in vegetables, even when cooked, but when you can, these are good sources.
- Calcium-fortified orange juice and other foods. Many products, in addition to orange juice, are now being fortified with calcium—bread, for instance. Look for labels on packaging that announce "calcium enriched" or "calcium fortified" and, if they meet the other requirements of your diet, add them to your shopping list.

■ Beans such as navy and pinto beans. Although beans are high in calcium, absorption of much of the mineral is hampered by other organic molecules present in beans such as phytates. Also, beans (as you know) produce a lot of gas and have a great deal of fiber. However, if you can tolerate them, they are very healthy foods for a number of reasons.

Trigger Foods

When you have an IBD flare, it is easy to believe that it is because of something you ate. You have gas and bloating and abdominal pain and that after all is where the food is. It didn't hurt before you ate, so it must be the food, right? While this sounds reasonable, it is only partly correct.

Keep in mind that IBD is an inflammatory disease in which your immune system attacks your intestine. What causes a flare is not fully understood. Certain foods—beans, for example—cause gas and bloating in most people, whether or not they have IBD. Likewise, a sudden large intake of sugar will often cause diarrhea. In essence, certain foods have inherent properties that determine how they are going to interact with the GI tract. The best example is a cut on your hand. You are not going to put salt on the cut, right? It will make the cut hurt worse. But it would not make the cut heal more slowly. That is what the wrong food can do: give you symptoms to make you feel worse but it is not making the inflammation worse. It is not surprising that they cause the same symptoms in people with IBD as they do for anyone. But for you, there's really no way of knowing whether it was the food, your immune system, or both that is behind your discomfort. It might be the early stages of a flare, or it might not.

A likely response to having a flare after consuming a suspect food is to eliminate that food from your diet. Unfortunately, that food may not be the cause, and then you have limited your diet unnecessarily. Over time, you may find that you have severely restricted your diet, even to the point of malnutrition.

A better approach is to keep careful records of what you eat. By comparing your intake over the course of several flares, you can begin to see if there are common triggers. If so, you can eliminate those for awhile and see if fewer symptoms occur. Finally, you can reintroduce the suspected food in small doses and see if symptoms return.

The main thing to remember is that everyone with IBD is unique in relation to the foods that seem to make a flare occur. Just because you have Crohn's disease does not mean that you have the same dietary intolerances as another person with Crohn's disease. The analogy for this is perfumes. You go to the department store, and there are hundreds available. What smells good on you may not smell good on your sister or best friend, because it has to do with personal body chemistry. The same holds true for foods and diets: it is not one-size-fits-all with global mandates for everyone with the same disease. In fact, your health care provider may tell you that if you have ulcerative colitis, it does not matter what you eat. What he or she really means is that it is unlikely that what you eat will contribute significantly to controlling the actual inflammatory process that is occurring. Again, there are inherent properties in foods that will give you GI symptoms, but that would occur in anyone, not just in someone with IBD. Your own experience is the best guide for what has an effect on you.

Reactions to Wheat Gluten and Other Foods

What is the role of wheat gluten in managing IBD? An autoimmune reaction to wheat gluten is called *celiac disease* or *celiac sprue* and is a condition different from IBD. It is characterized by an immune-mediated reaction at the lining of the small intestine that causes "rejection" of the food item containing gluten, which results in diarrhea, gas, bloating, and cramps. This is different from other kinds of food "allergies" that people can have. This reaction causes damage to the nutrient-absorbing villi that line the small intestine. Over time, nutrient deficiencies can occur as well as malnutrition because of this damage.

The treatment for celiac disease is total avoidance of items containing gluten, which includes all breads and products made with most grains. Unfortunately, gluten is a popular additive to many foods and even some medications and is difficult to avoid without being a food detective. People with IBD sometimes feel better when they take gluten out of their diet. That may be true, but it does not mean that they have celiac disease. When you take out such a common entity, it means you are eating more fresh items and preparing meals at home rather than eating out. This tends to be an overall healthier way to eat! However, taking gluten out of the diet does not cure IBD.

You may wonder whether you have been misdiagnosed with IBD and actually instead have a food allergy. There is certainly a lot we do not understand about the immune system and the way it interacts with the digestive tract, and it's impossible to tell someone with certainty that he or she isn't having some sort of allergic reaction to certain foods, in addition to having IBD. Proving the presence of a food allergy means systematically working your way through tedious elimination diets and careful reintroduction of individual foods to watch for a return of symptoms. A food allergy tends to be predictable once you find the culprit, because the absence of that item results in well-being and its reintroduction results in symptoms. Complete avoidance allows for healing and health. But we have not found such a straightforward link between any food and IBD. There are just so many different kinds of people who have IBD, with varied diets and sources of calories, that it seems very unlikely that we will find that a common dietary item is behind the symptoms.

Your Need for Glutamine

Keeping the cells that line your intestinal tract as healthy as possible is a major self-management goal in IBD. One of the ways of doing this is to keep those cells well fed, and their "food" of choice is an amino acid called glutamine. Glutamine should be of particular interest to you as someone who has IBD.

Glutamine is a major component of the protein we eat. It is also the most common amino acid in the body, especially in our muscle tissue and our blood. You know by now that, with the exception of alcohol, all foods that contain calories are composed of carbohydrates, fats, and proteins, either separately or mixed together in different proportions and different arrangements in different foods. That seems pretty simple to remember. However, each of these main categories is itself composed of different arrangements of their own primary ingredients: sugars and starches in carbohydrates, fatty acids in fats, and amino acids in proteins. There are 21 different kinds of amino acids from which proteins can be assembled, and each performs a slightly different function.

One of the functions of glutamine is to maintain the health of the cells that line the intestinal tract (the intestinal mucosa), which use it for fuel.[236–238] By keeping these cells well nourished, they can better fight off disease-causing organisms for the whole body. They also work to prevent "leaky gut," in which molecules from food or ingested toxins or bacteria leak into the blood from the intestine. There is also some evidence that these molecules can stimulate an immune response, initiating a flare of your IBD.

In addition to maintaining gut health, glutamine is helpful in restoring tissue damaged during an inflammatory episode. Fortunately, it is most abundant in foods that are well-tolerated during these times. The easiest way to get extra glutamine into your diet is to eat lots of the foods you already associate with protein—poultry, fish, and red meat. Beans and dairy products are also rich in glutamine but, because of high fiber content or lactose intolerance, are not appropriate during a flare or until your gut is recovered. Some vegetables and fruits are also rich in this amino acid. Glutamine in food is not known to affect people in a negative way. Glutamine in supplements is more concentrated and so you should be sure to talk with your health care provider about whether supplementation is appropriate for you.

Malnutrition in IBD

Unfortunately, it is common to see people with IBD who have malnutrition. Being malnourished does not necessarily mean being underweight. Malnutrition occurs when the internal nutrient supplies that your body needs to do its job properly are not adequate. This is most likely to happen when abdominal pain causes loss of appetite. And some people become afraid to eat or overly restrict their diets. As a result, poor intake comes at just the time when the intestine loses its ability to absorb nutrients and fluids, leading to vitamin and mineral deficiencies and weight loss.

How can you prevent or reverse malnutrition?

- Eat enough calories. Most adults with IBD require 25 to 35 calories per kilogram, or 11 to 15 calories per pound, of their healthy body weight.
- Eat several small meals throughout the day that, taken together over the course of the day, meet your nutritional requirements of calories, protein, vitamins, and minerals.
- If you really can't eat adequate amounts of healthy food, consider an oral nutritional supplement. A calorie-concentrated formula may be needed for those who require a large number of supplemental calories per day. These concentrated liquids usually have twice as many calories per ounce than regular ones.
- Consider vitamin/mineral supplementation, especially the following.
  - Folic acid. Taking sulfasalazine or methotrexate may alter folic acid absorption and metabolism, so supplementation is recommended with 1 mg per day. Folic acid also protects against colon cancer.
  - Vitamin D. Increased disease activity promotes deficiency and contributes to low bone mineral density and osteoporosis. In fact, vitamin D is the most common deficiency in Crohn's Disease. Recommended dosing is 800 to 1,000 IUs per day in pill or capsule form.
  - Vitamin B_{12}. Because the terminal ileum is the site of B_{12} absorption, if you have disease located in the ileum or have had resection of the ileum, you are at increased risk for B_{12} deficiency. Bacterial overgrowth also appears to increase the

risk. B$_{12}$ deficiency is most effectively treated with periodic injections, but some individuals do well with large doses of oral B$_{12}$ supplements. Some experts say that you need monthly shots, but others say that once every three months is sufficient.

- Zinc. Severe diarrhea, enteric fistulas, and moderate-to-severe disease activity can each result in deficiency. The recommended daily allowance is 15 mg per day, which is provided by many formulations of over-the-counter pills.

- Iron. Bleeding, lack of appetite, and decreased absorption all can lead to iron deficiency. It's common in IBD, so make sure your blood levels are monitored. Recommended supplementation for deficiency is 150 to 200 mg of elemental iron per day in addition to increasing your intake of iron-rich foods.

When You Can't Eat Food

You may have periods when you need supplemental nutrition because you're not eating enough to stay nourished or you're losing too much weight or just not gaining the weight that you need to stay healthy. When your health care providers talk about *enteral nutrition,* it means supplying calories directly to the GI tract. This can be in the form of supplements or specialized formulas that contain "predigested" nutrients so that your body does not have to work to break them down.[239, 240] They can be given via feeding tubes placed in the nose, stomach, or small intestine. In addition to supplementing eating, they can also be used as the sole source for nutrition when you can't eat at all or are very sick with severe disease activity. It can help. Studies have shown that nutritional therapy using enteral products may result in disease remission rates quite similar to when corticosteroids are used, perhaps because of the ability of the body to heal when rested in this manner.[241] However, very few people want enteral nutrition as the sole source of nutrition for very long.

Total parenteral nutrition (TPN) is utilized when the enteral route is not available or when absolute bowel rest is necessary and feeding via an IV is the only way to get nutrition. This is necessary when there is a prolonged bowel obstruction, a fistula between the intestine and skin, or very active disease that has not responded to other medical treatments.[242-244] There are few data exploring the effect of TPN on IBD as a treatment, although based on the studies that have been completed, TPN appears to have more of a benefit for people with Crohn's disease than ulcerative colitis. Complete bowel rest and thus the use of TPN becomes important when trying to heal fistulas caused by Crohn's disease. If you are in the hospital and unable to take in adequate calories, TPN is a part of the overall treatment plan for the short term.

Diets Specifically for IBD

You have probably wondered whether you should try one of the specific diets for treating IBD that are being promoted in other books. We are asked all the time about the "best" diet out there. One of the more popular diets is the Specific Carbohydrate Diet, as described in the book *Breaking the Vicious Cycle* by Elaine Gottschall. She claims that her diet, based on the theory that carbohydrates are the primary source for intestinal bacteria that contribute to IBD, cured her daughter's colitis. The diet consists of a grain-free, lactose-free, and sucrose-free regimen that prohibits:

- all grains, including corn, oats, and rice
- sugar, sucrose, fructose, and high-fructose corn syrup
- canned vegetables
- canned/processed meats
- starchy tubers (potatoes, yams, parsnips)
- bread, pasta, and other starchy foods
- milk, most milk products, and ice cream
- candy, chocolate, margarine, and ketchup

So, what is left to eat, you ask?

- fresh meat, poultry, fish, shellfish, and eggs
- fresh or frozen vegetables
- legumes (beans, lentils, peas)
- most hard cheeses
- honey
- most fruits and nuts
- coffee, tea, and juices with no additives

There are no data from scientifically conducted controlled studies to suggest that this diet works to treat or cure IBD. All the support you might read is in the form of testimonials from people who have followed the diet. Having read the book, I would comment that the diet is not harmful but is certainly not one that most people would be able to follow successfully. Almost all of the foods in the diet have to be prepared at home using flour made from almonds or other nuts and honey as the sugar source. Dr. Gottschall states in the book that the diet will not be successful unless you are "strictly adherent" to the diet, with no deviations. With those caveats in mind, I have no issue with you following this diet if you feel that it gives you some control over the state of your health. But please understand that there are no guarantees about what it will do for you.

The other popular books for healthy gut diets include a series of books based on eating for your blood type and *The Maker's Diet* by Jordan Rubin. *Eating for Your Blood Type* covers a variety of different conditions, not just IBD. That is one indication to be wary of the claims; how can a single type of diet help Crohn's disease, IBS, peptic ulcer, *and* diverticulitis? These conditions involve different mechanisms for their symptoms and anatomic abnormalities. The Maker's diet is specific to IBD and is built on a three-stage program that includes a restrictive diet as well as spiritual healing as taught in the Bible. I do not endorse any one particular diet because none have been shown to change disease in a significant number of patients. It seems I must continually point out that there are many different "miracle" diet programs out there. If one was truly the miracle cure, why would there be a continued market for the other books? Changing your diet to gain more control over symptoms and to improve your health are positive self-management measures but are not cures.

The following sample menus are for specific IBD situations. These are examples based on what we understand about IBD flares and the characteristics of specific foods and your need to avoid malnutrition. I encourage you to use these menus as starting places to experiment with what foods you can use to best manage your IBD.

During a Flare or When You Are Feeling Bad

This sample eating plan provides about 7 grams of fiber, nearly all soluble, over the course of a day.

Breakfast:
- ½ cup regular cream of wheat. Stir in ½ tsp. smooth peanut butter, ½ tsp. sugar or honey, and cinnamon to taste. Top with ¼ cup soy milk or cow's milk (if it doesn't bother you).
- ½ cup clear apple juice

Midmorning snack:
- 6 canned mandarin orange sections

Lunch:
- 1 cup chicken noodle soup with ¼ cup finely chopped canned carrots stirred in
- ½ slice white bread, lightly toasted, topped with sliced hard-boiled egg and "lite" mayonnaise
- 3 to 4 slices of canned peaches (not halves)

Afternoon snack:
- 3 saltines topped with tuna, mixed with small amount of mayonnaise or substitute. It is okay to use a small amount of onion powder for flavoring if it doesn't bother you.
- 4 ounces of purple or white grape juice

Dinner:
- 3 to 4 ounces of broiled salmon
- ½ cup boiled, peeled zucchini (no need to seed) with small amount of salt/pepper
- small boiled or mashed potato with skin removed, with ½ tsp. butter and small amount of salt/pepper
- ½ cup of applesauce

Evening snack:
- 2 crackers made with white flour topped with 1 tsp. smooth peanut butter on each
- ½ cup of apple juice

Substitutions: When you begin to get tired of these particular foods, start to make substitutions but do so without adding fiber or dairy. The exception to this rule is if dairy products do not normally bother you when you are not in a flare. Then it is okay to experiment with them during a flare. Just be aware that sometimes foods that you can tolerate at one time cannot be eaten without making your symptoms worse at another time. It will be very helpful to keep track of what you are eating, and how you are reacting to it, in a food diary so you can spot trends and stick with what works.

- Instead of cream of wheat, try cream of rice or a packet of plain instant oatmeal with no added flavorings or fruit pieces or, if you want to get back to dry cereals, try Rice Krispies.
- Instead of chicken noodle soup, try any broth: meat, poultry, fish, or vegetable. Substitute white rice or small pieces of boiled, skinless potato for the noodles. For added protein, stir a beaten egg into the hot broth with a fork or add very small pieces of lean, skinless cooked meat.
- Instead of apple or grape juice, use any kind of juice you like as long as it has no pulp.
- For fruit, try canned varieties of peaches, apricots, grapefruit, or pineapple in small amounts. Start with a few small pieces one

day then wait a day or two as you find your tolerance level to add any more. Fresh cantaloupe, watermelon, and honeydew melons have little fiber, mostly soluble, and are tolerated well.

■ Instead of mayonnaise, use any salad dressing you like, such as Miracle Whip, as long as it has no pieces of vegetable or herb particles in it. You can strain those bits out of a favorite bottled dressing with a coffee filter before using it. If you like, you can flavor your own oil and vinegar with herbs of your choice but strain it before using to remove the herb bits.

■ Instead of saltines or soda crackers, use any type of cracker made of plain white flour with no added fiber, bran, whole grains, or seeds. Oyster crackers or Carrs Table Water crackers are examples.

■ Instead of canned tuna, try canned salmon, any fish without bones, or smoked oysters. But you will probably do better without the more "stringy" shellfish such as fresh, smoked, or canned clams or shrimp.

■ Instead of broiled salmon, try a fresh or frozen fish fillet such as tilapia, cod, halibut, or whitefish without skin or bones. The breading may have preservatives or extra sodium in it, so try it without breading. Broil or steam until very soft. Canned fish is also acceptable.

■ For vegetables, try canned vegetables, specifically green beans, skinless and seedless tomatoes, tomato sauce or paste, or asparagus. Small amounts of finely chopped cucumber without skin or seeds are okay.

■ Instead of peanut butter, try any nut butter that has been very finely ground and has no "chunks" but use small quantities (1 to 2 tsp. at a time). Cashew or almond butter is often available in grocery stores.

When You Start to Feel Better

As your symptoms begin to subside, start reintroducing a small amount of fiber and a few of your favorite foods as long as they are low fiber and nondairy. The smartest way to do this is to change one meal or snack at a time and add it in small amounts.

For example, substitute the breakfast or dinner below for the one you have been using. On day 1, eat a half portion. If by the next day you have no adverse side effects, eat a half portion again on days 2 and 3. If, on the morning of day 4, you are still feeling well, start eating the full amount of the meal. If you are still doing fine after a week, substitute another meal or snack for the "eating during a flare" version. If you encounter problems, go back a step until you feel better. Then, try again, but instead of changing an entire meal or a snack at a time, change only one food.

It will help a lot if you write down what changes you make and how you feel after you eat something new. If you connect a particular food with unpleasant symptoms, eliminate that food for awhile until you feel completely healed. If that particular food is one of your favorites, try it again starting with a very small amount. You may be able to tolerate a little of it once every four or five days, and even though that is not as much as you might like, doing it this way will allow you to have it occasionally or on special occasions.

The "feeling better" sample menu below has a few more grams of fiber and a few more calories. But it's best to continue with small, frequent meals rather than eat too much at one time.

Breakfast:
- ¾ cup Special K cereal with ⅓ cup soy milk or cow's milk (if it doesn't bother you) and ½ tsp. sugar, if desired
- 1 peeled, ripe plum. Peeling is very important. Most skins contain insoluble fiber, which will make you worse. But the pulp contains soluble fiber, which should help you get better. Even skins that contain pectin, a soluble fiber, are tough and may be abrasive, so it is best to avoid them.

Midmorning snack:
- ½ slice white toast with 1 tsp. smooth peanut butter and a little clear jelly

Lunch:

- ½ cup pureed vegetable soup. Dilute a canned variety with water as directed and blend until smooth.
- Tuna "salad" on ½ piece white toast. Mix tuna with "lite" mayonnaise and a little onion powder and small amount of dill.
- 1 cup of watermelon chunks

Afternoon snack:

- ½ boiled skinless, boneless chicken breast dipped in a blend of soy sauce and either fresh ground or powdered ginger

Dinner:

- 3 to 4 ounces turkey breast
- ½ cup mashed potatoes with small amount of turkey gravy
- ½ cup canned green beans
- small piece of spice cake topped with small amount of powdered sugar

Evening snack:

- ½ cup applesauce with a bit of cinnamon, if desired
- ½ toasted white English muffin with 1 tsp. margarine or peanut butter

Substitutions:

- For juice, try any kind of fruit juice without pulp.
- For fruit, try any canned fruit without noticeably tough skins or any fresh melons.
- For bread, try any white bread or cracker—no whole grains.
- For cereals, try any kind with less than 2 grams of fiber and less than 6 grams of sugar in one cup. Examples are Rice Krispies, Corn Flakes, Crispix, Product 19, Special K, and Corn Chex. There are others, so read the labels.
- For vegetables, try any kind of canned vegetables without hard seeds or tough skins. *Do not* use corn or legumes, such as peas, kidney beans, navy beans, pinto beans, lentils, or chili beans.

- Instead of turkey, chicken or fish, try any tender, moist meat that does not have gristle or tough connective tissue.
- Instead of spice cake, try a soft cookie made with white flour or ginger snaps dipped in tea or milk.

Getting Back to Normal

If you have tolerated the addition of small amounts of fiber and sugar and larger portions without ill effects, you may begin to "normalize" your diet even more.

Breakfast:
- ¾ cup cooked instant oatmeal with 1 tsp. honey and ½ cup soy or rice milk or cow's milk (if it doesn't bother you)
- 4 ounces of clear juice

Midmorning snack:
- ½ banana
- ½ graham cracker with 1 tsp. smooth peanut or almond butter

Lunch:
- 1 cup egg-drop soup with oyster crackers. Stir a beaten egg into boiling chicken broth.
- Tuna sandwich on white bread. Mix 3 ounces tuna with mayonnaise or salad dressing and 1 large chopped lettuce leaf
- ½ peeled apple or 6 mandarin orange sections

Afternoon snack:
- Few ounces of pickled herring or smoked salmon on saltine crackers
- 4 to 5 peeled grapes

Dinner:
- 3 to 4 ounces of pressure-cooked or very tender, moist roast beef
- ½ cup mashed potatoes or white rice with a little margarine or gravy

- ½ cup very soft cooked broccoli or carrots
- ¼ ripe cantaloupe

When You Have Recovered from a Flare: Maintenance

Try these foods by adding them in small doses and one at a time. This sample menu has more protein and quite a bit of soluble fiber to provide the nutrients that will make your intestinal cells healthy and assist in their repair. Unless you are lactose intolerant, try yogurt, a form of dairy that is often tolerated, but do it carefully, a little amount at first, then larger amounts if you continue to feel well. It's important for you to continue to avoid large amounts of insoluble fiber.

Breakfast (2 options):
- Egg omelet with small amounts of well-cooked onion, garlic, tomato (seeds and skin removed), peeled zucchini or other summer squash, and/or chopped cooked spinach, kale, or chard
- 1 slice white toast with margarine and jelly, if desired
- ½ cup frozen hash browns cooked in small amount of olive or canola oil
- 2 to 3 ounces of cooked ham
- 4 ounces of apple juice

or

- 1 cup "instant" or "quick" oatmeal with 1 tsp. smooth peanut butter, ½ sliced banana, and ¼ to ½ cup skim cow's milk or soy milk
- 4 ounces of orange or grapefruit juice

Lunch:
- 1 cup canned tomato/vegetable-based soup or meat-based soup with ½ cup (per 2 cups liquid) added canned vegetables of your choosing (no corn or cooked dried beans)
- Chicken or turkey sandwich with 1 to 2 slices of white or seedless rye toast, mayonnaise or salad dressing, 1 lettuce leaf, and 1 slice of peeled tomato

- 4 to 6 sweet potato chips
- ½ orange with white membrane removed

Dinner:
- ½ baked marinated chicken breast
- ½ cup mashed winter squash
- ½ cup white rice
- ½ cup well-cooked or canned asparagus
- 6 ounces of low-fat, artificially sweetened yogurt without added fruit (flavorings okay)

Snacks:
- Smooth nut butters on white flour crackers (no crackers with whole grains or seeds)
- Applesauce
- Peeled, seedless fruits (no berries)
- Fruit juices, either clear or with small amounts of pulp
- V-8 or tomato juice
- Low-fat, artificially sweetened yogurt, but no more than 1 cup per day and only after testing with smaller amounts first
- Pickled herring, sardines, smoked oysters, smoked clams, fish pates on crackers made from white flour
- Gelatin desserts, plain or with pieces of canned, skinless fruits added
- Puddings made with soy or rice milk or skim cow's milk (if tolerated)
- Watermelon, cantaloupe, or honeydew melon

General Guidelines for Healthy Eating with IBD

- Use mostly canola and olive oil for salads, recipes, and cooking and eat fish often. The omega-3 fatty acids found in these oils and fish, shrimp, and other seafood suppress inflammation. It is possible to get omega-3 fatty acids from plant sources like walnut and flax seed oils, but doing so requires our bodies to perform a chemical conversion that is not done very effectively. Consequently, they are not major sources of omega-3 fatty acids and it's better to eat fish like herring, salmon, halibut, flounder, swordfish (but not for pregnant women due to mercury content), and pollack to suppress inflammation. Most salad oils except olive oil contain primarily omega-6 fatty acids, which actually promote inflammation, so avoid soy, safflower, corn, cottonseed, sunflower, and peanut oils.

- Eat small, frequent meals. You want to avoid getting too full or asking your digestive tract to process a lot of food at once. At the same time, you need additional calories and protein for repair of damaged tissues. By eating small amounts frequently, you meet those requirements without distending your gut and causing irritation such as bloating, cramps, and changes in bowel habits.

- Stay away from foods high in fat and/or sugar because both cause irritability of the GI tract because they cannot be digested all at the same time. You can feel bloated, full, cramping, and distended by meals high in these things. Fish oil is an exception to this rule.

- Drink a lot of fluids, primarily water. You need water to move fiber through your bowels.

- Learn to use a pressure cooker. You can make meats and vegetables very tender and break down the fibers so they are easier for your gut to tolerate.

11

Taking Charge of Your Lifestyle

Pain

Pain, as discussed in the other chapters as well, is a very broad topic and can come from many different sources. Certainly the concern will always be that pain is coming from active inflammation from within the GI tract. However, there are many other reasons to have pain, and it can sometimes be very difficult to manage. Sometimes patients feel uncomfortable discussing their pain with their physicians. At times, they feel judged, especially if their labs are normal and aren't "supposed" to be in pain or they are "supposed to be better by now." Physical pain is very hard to deal with emotionally—not just physically. People feel vulnerable and at the mercy of those treating them. The key is to have a real partnership with, not a dependence on, a health care provider that will allow you to work together to solve chronic pain issues.

One of the reasons it can be difficult to manage is because we don't have a good way of objectively measuring pain. What is very painful to one person is only slightly bothersome to someone else—we all have different pain thresholds. You may feel frustrated because your predominant symptom is pain, and your health care provider is telling you that "nothing is wrong." What that means is that he or she can't find anything abnormal on tests, but that doesn't mean you don't have pain. What will really help is to keep an accurate diary of your pain, as well as be as specific as you can about what you are actually experiencing and when. For example, is the pain all the time? Is it worse after meals, or at night? What makes it better? Is it always in the same place or does it move?

Some common reasons to have pain include active disease, obstruction, irritability of the GI tract, and side effects from medications. Other times the pain is coming from something totally unrelated to your IBD, perhaps the gallbladder, a peptic ulcer, or endometriosis. Remember, just because you have IBD does not make you immune to other conditions. I have missed the diagnosis of a ruptured tubal pregnancy because I was so focused on a patient's Crohn's disease.

Sometimes after a thorough work up for causes of pain (including blood and stool tests, X-rays and maybe even colonoscopy) there is no obvious explanation. Some causes to consider are again a side effect from a medication (antidepressants can cause abdominal pain), pain of the muscles of the abdominal wall (abdominal wall syndrome), early shingles, or neuropathic pain (pain that is originating from irritated nerve fibers along the wall of the bowel or inside the abdominal wall itself). This is sometimes called *visceral hypersensitivity,* where the nerves are inappropriately sensitive and tell the body there is pain when they really shouldn't be doing that. This may be harder to treat than other types of pain and needs a multipronged approach to manage. Withdrawal from narcotics can also cause rebound pain.

Pain can be managed in a lot of different ways. Some people unfortunately become addicted to narcotics because they need them at first and then take them for such a long time that their body gets used to them and have worse pain when they stop. Chapter 6 has information about pain relievers. One of the important things to keep in mind is that there are many times that pain cannot be completely obliterated, but the goal is to keep it at a minimum that allows for daily functioning. Only when a patient has very active disease or is obstructed, or there is another obvious mechanical abnormality is surgery the appropriate way to manage pain.

Stress

Stress falls into that odd category of hard to define, but you know it when you feel it. Stress can be positive, such as a child's wedding, or negative, such as being stuck in a traffic jam. Stress, simply defined, is deviation from the norm that you are powerless to avoid. It can be brief, such as worrying about missing a day of work due to illness, or chronic, such as having to deal with a critical boss each work day.

We all know that stress is bad for us and can take a toll on our bodies in different ways. Although stress does not cause IBD, it can certainly make it worse or even unmask it in someone who has not yet been diagnosed by increasing the symptoms so much that he or she seeks medical care.[245–249]

For me, the interesting thing is the connection between IBD, stress, and the immune system. We are just beginning to understand the relationship between the human immune system and the stress response. Because everyone is so different, it is difficult to scientifically test for the mechanisms by which "stress" affects the immune system and its function. Everyone deals with stress differently, and what is stressful to one person is a normal day to another. It is important to recognize what triggers your own personal stress response and deal with it. One can never totally avoid stress, but purposefully making choices to avoid excessive stress is always the best strategy.

Take the end-of-the-year holiday season, for example. Talk about stress! Even though holidays are supposed to be joyous, studies show that more people become depressed around the holidays than at other times of the year. There are many obstacles to enjoying yourself, and you definitely don't keep your normal routines. There is always temptation, with all the extra seasonal foods that become available, to eat more or try something unusual. This can be hard on your digestive system. Consider preparing for this time of year in terms of your schedule and diet as much as you can and don't stop taking your medications. There is no holiday from your need to keep inflammation at bay and your body in balance. This will help you avoid a flare. It probably won't surprise you to know that I get the largest number of calls from patients in distress around the holidays.

There is a misperception among both doctors and the public that people who are highly strung or have a "type A" personality are more at risk for IBD. This is just not true. People of all personality types, ethnicities, and cultures get IBD. Healthy, proactive techniques to relieve stress can be a means to control disease symptoms that seem to be driven by stress.

Sleep and Fatigue

It's easy to overlook your need for a good night's sleep and downplay its importance. But being well rested is central to being healthy. Experts agree that everyone should get 7 to 8 hours of sleep a night and that most of this time should be uninterrupted sleep. However, your sleep might be cut short or interrupted by diarrhea or pain. This can start a vicious cycle in which you are constantly ill because you cannot get adequate rest. I urge you to discuss persistent fatigue or excessive sleepiness with your health care provider. These can be a signal of ongoing inflammation or another condition, such as sleep apnea.

Some people use sleep aids because of their inability to fall asleep or to stay asleep. Others may use narcotics for this purpose. Most sleep aids will not interact with the medicines used to treat your IBD but can be addictive. It is important that you understand why you are not getting enough sleep, as these aids do not cure the problem. Melatonin is a natural agent that is a hormone that your body produces to help with the awake-sleep cycle in your brain. It is available quite widely in stores and pharmacies and might be a safer alternative than prescription pills.

Sometimes, fatigue is the only symptom of active inflammation, so you need to let your health care professional know about it so it can be treated. But, if your IBD seems to be under control and you are still really tired, then you deserve a workup to look for other causes.

Fatigue is one of those highly nonspecific symptoms. It often takes some digging to figure out why someone feels "tired all the time." Sure, having active IBD can wear you out, but I see many patients who are fatigued and aren't having an active bout of inflammation. Having IBD doesn't keep you from developing fatigue for other reasons, such as a medication side effect, depression, high blood glucose levels, or simply a lack of sleep.

Anemia is often undertreated in those with IBD, as health care providers just assume that anemia is normal in a patient with IBD, given that there is bleeding and impaired ability to absorb iron. By the age of 50, about 15% of the American population has a thyroid issue, generally underactive thyroid, and needs thyroid hormone replacement, which improves the ability to sleep through the night. Fatigue is the classic symptom of sleep apnea, a condition in which breathing is interrupted during sleep. This stopping and starting of breathing keeps waking the person up—even though he or she may not even realize it. People with depression may not feel "depressed" in the classic sense but can have pains that are otherwise not explained or chronic fatigue.

Tell your health care provider about it, and don't let your health care provider brush away this complaint. Once you find the cause of fatigue, it can be treated. Fatigue doesn't have to keep you from doing the things you want to and should be doing.

Smoking

If you have Crohn's disease and you smoke cigarettes, the most important change you can make to improve your health is to stop smoking. In the late 1980s, research began showing that smoking cigarettes increases both your risk and your family's risk of developing Crohn's disease and worsens the progression of the disease.[250-255] Even secondhand smoke increases the risk for Crohn's disease in the children of smokers. Women are particularly vulnerable. Several studies have shown that women smokers who have Crohn's disease need more steroids, have more surgery, have flares earlier, and have less of a response to medications like Remicade. As few as five cigarettes a day makes the disease worse, as does exposure to secondhand smoke.

Think about why you feel motivated to smoke. There are many ways to successfully quit smoking, some of which you may not have heard about, so ask your health care provider about your options. This is such an important part of managing Crohn's disease that I often dedicate a patient's entire clinic visit to a discussion about smoking cessation.

Strangely, ulcerative colitis occurs less often in people who smoke cigarettes. It is when they quit that they develop the disease or experience a flare. This has been so predictable that trials using nicotine have been done to simulate the effects that nicotine has on colitis.[256-259] These studies did not prove to be helpful to most patients. Smoking does not convey protection against developing colitis. Smoking has many ill effects, so I encourage all patients to kick that habit.

Physical Activity

Being physically active is important for the ongoing health of your entire body as well as your outlook. When your disease is active, you may not feel up to getting out of bed, let alone exercising. But when it's in remission, I encourage you to build a habit of regular physical activity. The benefits of regular exercise include a sense of well-being, stronger bones, and weight control, just to name a few.

For most people with IBD, the only restrictions on activity are what you impose on yourself. Physical activity tends to "rev up" the bowel, as you may have already noticed. Exercising in the middle of the day or at the end of the day can minimize the normal reflexes of the bowel that make it naturally more active in the mornings. Some of my patients tell me that they feel nervous when they don't know the exact location of a washroom, but others train for and run marathons or participate in long group bike rides. If having a bathroom close by is your concern, exercising at a gym or fitness club or at home may be the answer for you.

Everyone should engage in some kind of aerobic exercise—brisk walking, cycling, swimming, or group aerobics classes—on a regular basis, and having IBD does not change that. Find a few activities that you enjoy, and work on your strength and endurance. One of the recommendations I make to my patients who say they "don't have time to exercise" is to get a dog. A dog absolutely demands that you get some exercise, if it's only to take him or her around the block. A dog can be an excellent companion when you're not feeling well, too, and pets are well-known stress reducers.

Travel

When your disease is active, you may not want to even leave the house, let alone travel. However, it is not always practical to plan trips around flares. Here are some travel tips for your comfort and safety.

- Always make sure you have enough medication with you when you are away from home, even if you're only going to work.
- Check your schedule for intravenous therapy before making any travel plans.
- If possible, choose to travel so that you have control over your food and water supply and as much bathroom access as you need.
- When planning international travel, be sure to understand any vaccination recommendations and requirements as well as any epidemic alerts that have been issued. Because therapy for IBD usually includes steroids, immunosuppressants, or biologics, vaccines that are made from live viruses (that you have no way to fight off) can harm you. These include vaccines against polio, yellow fever, chickenpox, and rotavirus.

- Discuss your travel plans in advance with your health care provider, who may be able to recommend a colleague or medical center to contact in an emergency and nonprescription therapies for traveler's diarrhea or to prescribe antibiotics to take with you. Your health care provider can also write you a letter stating your need for an aisle seat on airplanes. If you are traveling to a place that requires proof of vaccination and you have not been vaccinated because of the medications you are taking, then a letter from your doctor stating this is required.
- In addition to your medications, consider packing your own toilet paper or wipes in your airline carry-on luggage.
- Having an "emergency travel kit" may also give you peace of mind. Include a change of underwear, disposable panties or liners, toilet wipes or cream that can be used on toilet paper (like Balenol), and perhaps a roll of your favorite type of toilet paper.

Ally's Law is a law that first passed in the Illinois Senate. It was championed by a little girl from Chicago who was turned away from the employee washrooms at a clothing store when she had an urgent need to evacuate. She proceeded to have an embarrassing accident and was infuriated. The law grants people with a medical need access to washroom facilities from stores and merchants that otherwise don't offer public services. You can obtain a card to carry in your wallet that essentially acts as a "Free Pass" by contacting your local Crohn's and Colitis Foundation chapter or printing one off the internet at www.myibd.org.

Working

Having IBD means there is a good chance you will miss some work time due to disease flares, hospitalizations, and doctor's appointments. There are laws in place to prevent discrimination in the workplace due to chronic illness, but these laws affect employers in different ways. My advice is to not rely on yourself to figure this out—consult with an attorney to understand your legal rights. In general, employers must make accommodations for an employee with physical disabilities who is otherwise competent to fulfill a position. Before accepting a job, understand what will be expected of you and how the job may be modified if necessary to fit your needs. Get the advice of your legal counsel as to the correct time to introduce the discussion with an employer or potential employer about your IBD.

Only you can decide if and when to tell your boss or colleagues about your colitis or Crohn's disease. In a supportive work environment, people with IBD might be able to tell their bosses and coworkers about the struggles they endure and the accommodations they need. However, the world is not always sympathetic to people with illnesses, and it is very important to use common sense when deciding to whom, when, and how you disclose information about your condition.

With regard to your employer, try to predict how accommodating and compassionate he or she may be based on interactions with other colleagues who have faced health challenges. Have others been treated with understanding and flexibility? Most employers generally want their employees to be happy, because it maximizes productivity. Therefore, some of them may be willing to make necessary accommodations to assist with IBD challenges.

Colleagues may sometimes be a better choice than the boss if you need people to "lean on" at work. They also have a boss to answer to and may therefore be more understanding. With colleagues as well, however, you may want to use caution. Some colleagues may be generally supportive of one another. Others may gossip about each other to try to get ahead. If you're looking for support, consider choosing colleagues who have demonstrated good character in the past.

Also, remember that because most people have no preconceived ideas about what IBD means to an individual, what you say and how you say it will make all the difference. If you choose to disclose, be honest and clear about your illness and needs, and do so in a calm way. If you are very emotional in your presentation, people are more likely to be concerned that IBD will have a negative impact on your work. If you present your illness as a challenge that you rise to but still need some accommodations, people are less likely to see it as a potential barrier to your productivity and are more likely to assist.

So, what's the bottom line? If you trust the people you work for and with, it may be helpful to tell them about your IBD and ask for the assistance and accommodations you need.

- If you need to tell your boss, explain your illness in a calm, professional way.
- Be clear about the accommodations you need, such as a work space that is close to the bathroom.
- When considering job opportunities, keep your IBD in mind and choose a job that has some schedule flexibility.
- During flare-ups, request assignments that do not require long periods of time away from bathroom facilities.

These days, many jobs can be done from home or work hours can be arranged to be flexible. But there may be times when your priority is to get your health back on track and taking short-term disability from work can be the appropriate way to do this. Short-term disability periods tend to be about 3 months long, which is about the right amount of time it can take to focus on your health and get your disease under control. Permanent disability is an option if your disease symptoms are so unpredictable that trying to hold down even a part-time job is difficult. The Crohn's & Colitis Foundation of America is an excellent resource for help with determining whether disability is right for you (www.ccfa.org).

Useful Web Sites

The Internet can be both a helpful and harmful place to get information. The kind of information you can get from a Web site is only as good as its sources. Some sites are run by the government, others by organizations that want to give out accurate information, and still others are set up by pharmaceutical companies and, while helpful, can be slanted toward one product or another. Other sites are from organizations that have no vested interest in any one treatment or another and want to help as many people as possible.

A partial list of helpful Web sites is listed below. This is not inclusive but a good place to start for additional information.

- www.ccfa.org: The Crohn's & Colitis Foundation of America
- www.myibd.org: The Foundation for Clinical IBD
- www.ibdsf.com: The IBD Support Foundation, an organization that provides support programs by age and for parents
- www.j-pouch.org: For patients with J pouches
- www.clinicaltrials.gov: Where all clinical trials must be posted
- www.nih.gov: National Institutes of Health
- www.acg.gi.org: American College of Gastroenterology
- www.gastro.org: American Gastroenterological Association
- www.wecareinibd.org: We Care in IBD, an organization of women dedicated to the field of IBD
- www.uoa.org: The United Ostomy Association, where you can find out more about stomas and their care

12

Growing Up with IBD

Tyler had always been the "runt" of the class. He really never complained of anything, but there were days where he just could not keep up with the other kids on the playground. When he reached sixth grade, his parents felt that there may be something wrong. It was discovered that Tyler was anemic and iron deficient. Tyler denied ever seeing blood in his stools and didn't really complain of pain. However, he had learned to stay away from fried foods because they made him feel "bad." A CT scan revealed that a portion of his small intestine was inflamed, and a colonoscopy with biopsies revealed the diagnosis, Crohn's disease. Tyler started therapy with azathioprine and a multivitamin, both taken once a day, and he started to gain weight and had lots more energy.

Have you just learned that your child has IBD? You may be relieved to know what has been causing his or her symptoms but saddened because you and your child have now entered an unknown world. It is

189

difficult to stay calm and focus on learning the ways of this new world when you are wondering if there was something you could have done to prevent your child's IBD. Please don't spend much of your energy on feeling guilty. Research has shown us ways to manage IBD but not how to prevent this autoimmune disease. Autoimmune diseases like IBD seem to have both a genetic component and an environmental trigger, but the trigger or combination of triggers may be unique to the child.

It's natural for you to have questions, concerns, and even fears. There are other parents and children looking for answers and support, just as you are. You might be surprised to learn that about a quarter of the people who have IBD—estimated to be 1 million in this country—are younger than age 18. Children and teens have the same symptoms and mostly the same issues with IBD as adults do, but there are key differences. One of the biggest challenges is the relatively small number of pediatric gastroenterologists in the United States available to focus on the special care of this unique group.

The most common age at diagnosis is 12 and a half years, but children as young as 3 develop IBD.[260–264] In the preschool years, ulcerative colitis is as common as Crohn's disease. However, this shifts with age, and more school-age children develop Crohn's disease than ulcerative colitis, by approximately 3 to 1.

Developing a chronic disease at the age of 12 is a big deal.[265–267] Most children at this age are very self-conscious about their changing bodies and challenged by the rising hormone tides that go with the teen years. They are more awkward and off-balance physically and emotionally than they have ever been in their lives. As they move from elementary school to middle or high school, they feel the desire to *not* be seen as different from everyone else. What a time to add a chronic disease with symptoms that deeply embarrass and invasive but necessary medical tests and treatments! My heart goes out to each one of my young patients— and to you, their parents.

And then, I realize how strong and capable my young patients are. I have seen what this disease has taught them about themselves. Your bewildered children will find resiliency in themselves and maybe even humor in their situation. These are valuable traits to have when saddled with a chronic disease, which can't be cured and must be managed by your child working with health care providers. Consider that your child has the power to decide when to take his or her medications and what to eat. Our children get to decide whether they want to take good care of themselves, but they will always need your support and encouragement, and most of all, your hugs when all the right choices don't keep the illness in remission. We cannot manage IBD perfectly, and letting go of perfectionism might be a step in the right direction. Your role as parents? Cheerleaders!

Another step in the right direction is to acknowledge both your own and your child's feelings as they arise. Give the feelings "a place to sit at your table," and keep the conversation going. That will give you a way to acknowledge the new facts of life in your household and figure out the best way for your family to live with them. After all, a chronic illness affects everyone in the family in one way or another. You'll have to work together to define the "new normal" in your lives.

What Caused Your Child's IBD

As I wrote in Chapter 1, we don't know exactly why someone develops IBD, but it's under active investigation. There seems to be a genetic component, although any particular gene or combination of genes has not been definitively identified as the cause. Here are some facts:

- Just 30% of those diagnosed have a family history of some type of IBD.
- The chance of passing IBD along to a child is low, roughly 3% to 7%.
- If both parents have IBD, the chance of their child developing IBD increases to 45%.

Some have blamed the development of Crohn's disease on childhood vaccinations, similar to the thinking that vaccines increase the risk of autism, but the research does not support these ideas.

Growth and Development

Growing is the primary activity of childhood, and it requires a lot of energy, all fueled by food. So, it's especially tough to deal with a gastrointestinal illness when you're young. It is easier to notice when children are having difficulty absorbing nutrients because they grow and change so quickly, compared with adults. Failure to grow is often the first symptom we see, even before the GI symptoms that lead to an IBD diagnosis. It's not normal for children to lose weight, but this is a typical problem for the children I diagnose with IBD.

Crohn's disease seems to pose a bigger challenge to growth than ulcerative colitis. About a third of children have "failure to grow" when they are diagnosed with Crohn's disease, whereas only about 10% of children diagnosed with ulcerative colitis are classified this way. The most common cause of growth failure is malnutrition from absorbing too few calories, which points to issues with the small intestine. A child with ulcerative colitis who also has failure to grow needs to be thoroughly examined with a scope as well as X-rays for possible involvement of the small intestine in his or her disease as a source of this growth failure.

Malnutrition and failure to grow can lead to slower than normal development of puberty. These can be reversed if the growth plates in the bones have not fused shut, which was the case for Tyler. This usually happens around age 15, and Tyler had just turned 12 at diagnosis. For Tyler, we concentrated on treating the underlying inflammation as well as supplementing his diet with nutrients that were depleted, and this helped greatly to bring on growth spurts and ensure proper maturation through the phases of puberty. Tyler's parents worked hard to balance his treatment while keeping his routine as normal as possible, so that the emphasis was not put on the disease, but on Tyler and his ability to get past this.

How IBD Is Different for Children and Teens

The nature of IBD is different in children than in adults.[264] We tend to see more inflammation in the upper parts of the digestive tract in children, meaning the jejunum, stomach, and esophagus. This translates into potentially different symptoms than in adults. Inflammation in more of the small intestine will lead to more vague abdominal pain, stomach inflammation can lead to nausea and vomiting, and inflammation in the esophagus leads to trouble swallowing. If your child is diagnosed with either ulcerative colitis or Crohn's disease, it's important for the gastroenterologist to investigate the entire GI tract for any evidence of disease in more "unusual" places.

Crohn's disease in those younger than age 20 historically tends to be a more aggressive disease, involving more surgeries because the disease does not respond as well to medications, which we call *medically refractory*. What this means is that the usual medicines we use to treat adults don't seem to work for children. One of the ways that we can look for "aggressive" IBD—disease that may require stronger medications earlier in the disease course—is with blood tests that look for certain proteins (markers). We know of four different markers that are associated with the presence of IBD. Research has shown that children with more of these markers and at higher concentrations tend to have more aggressive disease than those who have no markers or have markers at low concentrations.[268] Children with IBD that is wide-ranging in the digestive tract or highly inflamed need to be treated aggressively, using immunomodulators from the start of therapy. Children who are started on steroids risk steroid dependency and failure to grow because of the length of time on steroids that is required to calm the disease.

Another major concern is the increased risk of colorectal cancer that is associated with having the disease for more years (see Chapter 8). This is why we need to be vigilant in screening for cancer at ages earlier than normal. Specifically, developing ulcerative colitis before age 15 is a known risk factor for the development of colon cancer well before the age of 50, supposedly because of the longer duration of disease. We have two ways to fight this increased risk. First, because therapy with 5-ASA seems to offer protection against colon cancer, this therapy is preferred and should begin right away. Also, your child needs regular screening colonoscopies: at diagnosis, after 8 years if he or she has extensive colitis, and after 10 years for left-sided colitis. This is the same schedule as adults with IBD.

Treating IBD in Children and Teens

Tiffany was diagnosed with ulcerative colitis at age 7. From the beginning, her parents tell me, she refused to take her medications and was "difficult." Tiffany denied that she had anything wrong with her. She hid her medicines under the bed instead of taking them. She would minimize her symptoms, but her parents said that she would spend hours in the bathroom in the morning before school and then after school. Tiffany refused to take lunch to school with her and told her parents that she was not hungry during the day. When she entered high school, her parents were concerned that she would develop an eating disorder and thought that she should be seen by a gastroenterologist who cares for adults. That's when I met Tiffany and had a chance to talk with her without her parents present.

Tiffany told me that the medicines she was prescribed tasted "icky" and had to be taken too many times per day. She felt alone, as she was an only child, and thought her parents focused "way too much on my colon." She had never met anyone else with ulcerative colitis. I suggested that she have her medicines changed to twice daily and think about spending a week at the Crohn's & Colitis Foundation camp to meet other kids like her. For Tiffany, that week was a life-changing, heartening experience. She has been at the camp every summer since and later became a volunteer, which has piqued her interest in pursuing a career in nursing to help kids with chronic illness.

The goals of IBD treatment are essentially the same for children and teens as for adults with IBD: control active inflammation and prevent complications. Our first line of therapy for those with mild-to-moderate ulcerative colitis and some of those with Crohn's disease is a 5-ASA medication. Those children with Crohn's of the small bowel or colon may have a response to 5-ASA if the disease is mild. However, most children with Crohn's disease will require medications stronger than 5-ASA to control the disease. A child who continues to have the symptoms that led to the diagnosis in the first place is probably not going to get the best long-term treatment by staying on 5-ASA.

Immunomodulators, such as 6-mercaptopurine, azathioprine, and methotrexate, are very effective therapies in children, as in adults.[269–271]

These are used to help avoid or wean off of steroids just like in adult patients. They are also the next step if 5-ASA medications don't work or stopped working. Infections are more common in children taking immunosuppressants, and schools are where infections tend to be shared quite readily among classmates. Watch your child to catch any developing infection early and encourage hand washing and other behaviors that will protect against infections. All immunosuppressed patients should receive an annual flu shot, but children on immunomodulators should not receive any live vaccines, such as polio or chicken pox vaccine. This is because a live vaccine is designed to purposely give the patient a little dose of the disease so that the body can build a defense against it. If you are immunosuppressed, then introducing an infection will just lead to a worsening infection and not necessarily immunity down the line.

Remicade is used to treat severe Crohn's disease in children because it has very high response rates and avoids the use of steroids.[272–279] In addition, growth rates with Remicade are much higher than when young patients are treated with steroids.[280] There are also smaller studies with the other biologics, Humira[281] and Tysabri.[282] Deciding to use a biologic is a big step, because you need to take it consistently. Chapter 6 explains why this is so. Another thing to know is that, to date, 14 young patients between the ages of 12 and 32 who had received Remicade in combination with azathioprine or 6-mercaptopurine have developed a rare T-cell lymphoma.[283–287] Most were males, but then the vast majority of those who have this type of lymphoma and Crohn's disease during the past 100 years were male. Because of the sudden increase in the numbers of patients with this rare tumor, we no longer use this combination of medications and instead treat with Remicade alone. Trials are underway for Remicade in children with ulcerative colitis as well as the other biologic agents.

In addition to controlling IBD with medications, we pay close attention to your child's growth. If your child is not growing as expected, nutritional supplementation becomes an important part of the treatment. This does not necessarily mean a special diet; we tend to use high-protein or high-calorie supplements, including protein shakes, Pediasure, and even tube feeding at night for extra calories. Although they are often used, steroids can significantly slow down a child's growth. Therefore, your child's IBD should not be controlled by using steroids between flares. If steroids are needed to treat flares, they are for short-term use only—no more than a few weeks.

When a child needs surgery, the surgical approaches to Crohn's disease and ulcerative colitis are similar to those in adults. There are specialized pediatric surgeons who operate on children and usually will care for them until the age of 18. If your daughter needs to have her colon removed because of ulcerative colitis, have a discussion with her doctors about safeguarding her future fertility. As discussed in Chapter 13, the J pouch procedure is associated with a decreased fertility rate in about 50% of females.[288] Although this may not be a concern when your daughter is 8 years old, it certainly will be when she is older.

Remember that what and how your child eats can determine how well she or he copes with IBD. Meeting with a nutritionist skilled in IBD can help you better understand your child's nutrition needs and result in meal plans designed to meet those needs. For a week or so in advance of your visit, keep a daily food diary to gather the information that will be most useful to the nutritionist, who needs an idea of what kind of foods your child is served at home and his or her personal likes and dislikes.

Monitoring IBD in Children and Teens

Laboratory testing, endoscopy, and X-rays are the cornerstone to diagnosis and assessment of IBD. However, we take some important aspects into consideration with pediatric patients. Computed tomography (CT) scans should be used only when necessary in children to minimize their exposure to radiation over their lifetime.[289–292] More and more often, MRIs, which do not involve ionizing radiation, are being used along with other types of noninvasive testing. For instance, a special kind of X-ray study called a white blood cell or "tagged white cell" scan can evaluate the presence of inflammation in the small intestine. Stool tests that look for certain proteins—lactoferrin and calprotectin are the two most commonly measured proteins—can reveal active inflammation when there is a question about it. These noninvasive tests can help us avoid having to put your child through an endoscopy, because young patients have this done under general anesthesia, not just conscious sedation as with adults. General anesthesia is used up to around age 15, but it depends a lot on the gastroenterologist, the practice patterns for that part of the country, and parental and patient preferences. Even if your child can't express it, he or she may fear an invasive procedure, and the preparation for a colonoscopy is not fun, either. Video capsule endoscopy, the "camera pill," is not yet well enough studied to be used in children.

Another type of test your child may need is X-rays to determine bone growth. Bone density scans done in adults may not be accurate in children. A plain X-ray of the arm can provide information about the child's growth potential when compared with his or her chronological age.

The blood protein tests used for diagnosis can also be helpful in monitoring your child's condition. Children with particularly aggressive disease have multiple markers present, four of which are currently being studied, and they appear in very high concentrations. It would make sense, then, to use these markers to predict the progress of the disease in children. The markers appear to be most helpful in those children with disease in their small intestine. The more markers present, and the higher their concentration, the more aggressive the therapy up front should be. But, it's important to put these markers into the context of the overall clinical picture. We must consider, for example, what the child eats, whether there is secondhand smoke in the home, and how well the child gets along with other family members. These are all factors that will have an impact on how active the disease is: food may make gastrointestinal symptoms worse, secondhand smoke makes Crohn's disease worse, and a stressful family life will affect the course of the disease.

The Importance of Staying on the Medications

It would appear to be easy to just take your medications on time every day. But all sorts of things can interfere with your child's desire to follow the doctor's guidance: how sick he or she is, how well the family supports her, how sympathetic the doctor is, and so on.[293] It's so tempting to quit taking the medications when IBD is in remission; after all, your child feels better and wants to be like everyone else, plus there are often undesirable side effects. But there are other reasons that would make a child resist staying on his or her medications. Perhaps the child is being teased about being sick or different. Maybe your family is embarrassed by your child's condition and wants to hide it, and the medications, from others. Maybe the medications are causing your family financial difficulty. Children are very sensitive to such issues. Maybe your teenager is rebelling against the physician's orders. All sorts of factors influence how well a patient follows the doctor's advice.

One way to deal with this is to be a good role model. Children will emulate the attitudes and health behaviors of the adults who surround them. Everyone has personal challenges to face, so perhaps you can show your child a consistent, healthy approach to something that's a chronic issue for you, like quitting smoking, weight loss, or being physically active each day.

Ask your child's health care providers to minimize the pill count or simplify the timing of doses so that pills don't need to be taken at school. If your child is permitted to carry his or her own medications at school, maybe he or she will want to keep them in an Altoids tin. One of my middle school patients did this so that taking her medicines just looked like she was having breath mints. Be sensitive about whether your child has a hard time swallowing pills or capsules; perhaps taking them with food works best. Another idea is to build a routine for the pill taking times that has everyone taking something, even a multivitamin, so the child with IBD is not alone.

Fitting in with IBD

We want the best quality of life for our young people with IBD, which includes a happy life. Children with IBD strive so hard to "fit in" and not to be different from their peers. The pressure of keeping such a secret can be so hard to live with, but it is uncommon for children with IBD to tell other children about their illness or other chronic diseases because they feel they will be teased or rejected. A sympathetic teacher could include a lesson on IBD to raise the awareness of other students without singling out your child, but you also run the risk of triggering the bathroom humor of many children, and embarrassing your child even further. It takes a balanced, calm approach to teach children about this disease. Your child's teachers should be able to help you evaluate the maturity and kindness of your child's classmates and predict how they will handle the information. Certainly, your child should think about adding best friends to the "support team."

What cannot be hidden are the esthetic and emotional side effects of certain medications, steroids in particular. The weight gain, "moon" face, and irritability that are typical of chronic steroid use can significantly affect how well your child gets along with family and friends, at home and at school. Fortunately, the other medications we use do not affect the appearance or emotional stability of a child.

Pay attention to your child's state of mind. Just as in adults, depression and anxiety can be common in children with IBD. We don't often think of children being depressed, but this disease provides them with so many challenges. Watch for signs of depression or anxiety in your child, especially if he or she has bodily complaints out of proportion to his or her IBD if it seems to be in remission. Missing a lot of school because of flares and hospitalizations can have an impact on your child's school performance and how classmates relate to him or her. You cannot control how often your child must be absent, but this will draw attention and curiosity from the other children. Does your child get special treatment from teachers? Other children can resent this if they don't understand what is going on—and it's very difficult for someone without the disease to fully understand what it requires.

Perhaps seeing a counselor as a family will provide a supportive place to identify and talk through issues that may be holding back your child's health. A psychosocial evaluation for your child and your family can be an important part of the overall management of his or her IBD. Pediatric IBD centers often include visits to a social worker or counselor along with visits to physicians, because our minds and emotions also are affected by IBD as well as bodies. These visits are a vital part of overall care.

Consider finding a peer support group that can help your child better understand how to deal with having IBD and find the motivation to do all that is required. Support groups and national camp programs, such as Camp Oasis, can play a very important role in helping your child and your family cope with IBD and even improve everyone's relationships and behavior. Teens, especially, may acquire new negotiation skills and feel empowered by taking better care of themselves.

It is important to remember that this is your child's body and your child's disease. Even if he or she is only 8 years old, your child is capable of helping with and even taking responsibility for parts of his or her health care. Believe that your child has what it takes to manage this disease, and communicate your belief to your child and the rest of your family. Children are quite resilient, and when they are treated with respect and dignity, they can be some of the most intelligent and inspiring patients I have. I am often humbled by the maturity and insight of my patients, some of whom have been dealing with this disease since early childhood.

Practical Advice about Common Parental Issues *by Marci Reiss, LCSW*

Who Gets to Know?

Speaking about your child's disease with others may seem like a simple issue, but there is actually much to consider before relaying information to others. There are many reasons why parents have discussions with others about their child's new diagnosis. First, most parents are understandably very emotional and have countless questions regarding the impact the illness is going to have on their child and their families. One common way for parents to begin doing their research is by speaking with others—for names of physicians and hospitals and to gain a general picture of what may be in store for their child and family. Additionally, because health is a very emotional issue, parents often talk to people because they are upset, and it is a common way of reacting to problems.

Sometimes, parents are so caught up in their own emotions and concerns, they do not think about the fact that what they are discussing is their children's private body parts and private bathroom habits. Their children, however, generally do not respond favorably to their family and friends finding out about their disease and their bowel habits. An effective approach is to discuss with your child who should know and respect his or her request. Imagine how you would feel if your child went to school and shared with friends that Mom spent hours in the bathroom with bloody diarrhea!

Ask Them How They Are Feeling—Once a Day!

Due to great concern, we ask our children how they are feeling many times throughout the day. They have already been told they have a disease, and frankly, most of them would like to forget about it. Children are forced to think about being different and having a disease every time they go to the bathroom and every time they take their pills. Between those two things alone, they are already thinking about their disease about five times a day at a minimum. That doesn't include every time they need to go to the doctor, have labs drawn, and so forth. Every time parents ask how they are feeling, they are once again forced to think about it. I recommend that parents establish limits of inquiry with their children: tell your child that one parent will ask once a day in order to not cause frustration and that your child gets to pick the time. In exchange, the child needs to be totally honest about what is going on in his or her body. Sometimes, they are so afraid of the repercussions of their symptoms, such as more medicine or more doctor visits, they don't share all the information. And of course, make sure your children know that they are welcome to raise the issue of their disease or ask questions at any time.

Medication Compliance

In running parenting groups for children with IBD, I have heard parents say countless times that they are so grateful that their children take their medications regularly and "it's not an issue for us," only to find out that in the next room, their children are telling their group facilitators that they have tossed, flushed, hidden, or even fed to the family dog their medications for the last two weeks! I would venture to say that almost all children become noncompliant with their medications at some point during their teenage years. Typically, it is when they are feeling well and naïvely think that a few weeks off isn't a big deal.

Unfortunately, I have also seen those same teens end up missing prom night or the school play and even ending up in surgery due to noncompliance. Because the stakes are so high, I encourage parents to actually watch their children take their meds. This needs to be done with great tact and sensitivity. In a nonchalant manner, parents should establish a morning or nightly routine (or both, depending on when the child needs to take the medication) and just spend some time with the child while they take their meds—even if it is just a minute or two. Some children will respond with comments such as, "you don't trust me!" I encourage parents to explain that it is not a matter of trust; instead, it is just that taking medication for an illness every day would be hard for anyone, and you would like to support them and be there with them during that difficult part of their day. Throwing in a favorite drink such as lemonade or chocolate milk is also helpful in sweetening the whole experience.

Guiding Children along Their Journey to Independence

Adolescence is a natural progression of children growing into independent adults. During that time, parents gradually lessen their involvement in the decisions their children make. For example, although parents are more likely to be involved in structuring their children's activities when they are younger, teenagers progressively make more and more of their own decisions regarding who they are spending their time with and what activities they are engaging in. This is a very healthy and natural process in which children grow into autonomous adults.

When a disease is thrown into the picture, parents have less ability to let go. They naturally are thrown off balance and try to tighten their grip on their children so they can protect them from their frightening new realities. Unfortunately, this can have a detrimental impact. Additionally, although healthy children generally are striving for independence and the ability to make their own decisions and choices, children who have been given a diagnosis of IBD have very often also been traumatized by pain or hospitalizations and medical procedures. This typically stifles their desire for independence and makes them regress into a more dependent state.

One of the ways parents can really assist their children in resuming their journey to adulthood is by allowing them to "take ownership" of their disease. Depending on their age and maturity level, children need to begin by speaking for themselves at their doctor's visits. Although this may sound obvious, many parents answer basic questions for their children, including "how are you feeling?" or "how many bowel movements are you having a day?" It is imperative to allow children to begin to speak for themselves. Even young children can answer simple questions and very often know the answers better than their parents; after all, the symptoms are occurring in their bodies! By the later teenage years, children should be encouraged to fully speak for themselves and even have their parents wait in the waiting room while they have their appointment.

IBD at School

There are many difficulties in adjusting to life with IBD as an adolescent. One of the main challenges is how to deal with IBD at school. For some lucky ones, it is rarely an issue, and most bathroom activity occurs early in the morning or after school. Most, however, need to figure out how to take medications at school without drawing too much attention, how to navigate making it to the bathroom in time or going in the middle of class, how to deal with homework when they are exhausted in the evenings, how to explain missed absences, and much more.

I recommend that prior to the school year, parents meet with teachers and make them aware of the student's disease and symptoms so that they may be supportive of the child in school. For example, teachers will often allow students with IBD to leave class without asking permission, so they can use the bathroom whenever necessary, with the understanding that the student will not abuse the privilege. In situations where the school or teachers are not cooperative and understanding, I recommend the implementation of government programs, such as a 504 plan, which is part of the Americans with Disabilities Act. Each 504 plan is individualized to the specific student's needs. It outlines the modifications and accommodations necessary for the particular student so that he or she has the opportunity to perform at the same level as peers. For students with IBD, these accommodations might include such things as bathroom access whenever the student needs it, freedom to use staff bathrooms to increase privacy, exemptions from certain physical education activities when the student does not feel well, extra time to complete assignments if the student is not well, or allowing for tardiness in the morning, when disease is often more active. The 504 plan is tailored to the individual and often gives the student a sense of comfort knowing that the disease will not hamper his or her ability to succeed in school.

Swallowing Pills: Practical Ways to Make It Easier

If you take a close look at how children eat, you will notice that most kids do not chew their food well. In fact, you can often hear parents saying to younger children, "Take smaller bites and chew!" Softer foods such as macaroni and cheese or vegetable soup really get swallowed without much chewing. This idea is important to remember if your child is struggling with swallowing pills.

Most likely, if there is difficulty with swallowing food, the child is simply afraid, not just of the pill swallowing, but about all of the changes and new frightening experiences that he or she is going through. Let your child know that you understand that all these changes are scary and that pills can be tough to take—even for grownups—and sometimes they leave a bad taste in the mouth. However, the medicine is a big part of what is going to make your child well, and the more the child sees pills as what is going to make them feel well again, the better.

Try not to pressure your child with regard to pills. The more stressed out you are, the more stressed they will be and the less successful at swallowing. Show them how they can eat mouthfuls of food (macaroni is really great for this) without chewing: they are swallowing food whole, and macaroni noodles are larger than most IBD pills. If necessary, tell your child that you're going to put one of the pills inside a tube-shaped noodle and to just eat the macaroni. This can be very successful, especially if you can distract the child and discuss something more pleasant as they are eating mouthfuls of food.

The most important part to remember is when there is difficulty with taking pills, the more relaxed and calm you are, the better. Your child will get there. Over time, even the ones who struggled with pill swallowing at the beginning become pros at taking several large pills at a time.

13

Sex, Fertility, and Pregnancy

So many visits with your health care providers are all about managing your IBD that you may not find time to discuss other important matters, such as intimacy. You may feel awkward discussing sex anyway, but it is often more difficult to do with someone you think may not understand or be sympathetic to your situation. Some of my patients feel comfortable enough to ask questions about engaging in sexual intercourse. I can assure them that, for almost everyone with IBD, this activity will not cause any undue stress on your disease and may actually make you feel more normal. For many people, sex plays an important role in creating a sense of well-being.

Engaging in physical intimacy also brings fears of incontinence or needing a washroom at an inopportune time and self-consciousness about changes in your appearance due to the disease or cosmetic side effects from steroids or surgery. You also may be dealing with fatigue, pain, and frequent bowel movements. You cannot get help for any of these issues if you don't talk to someone about them. Women may talk with their gynecologists, but because a fistula in the vaginal area is hardly ever seen on a physical exam, it may be hard for the gynecologist to make recommendations that address IBD issues. It is also important to remember that body parts and areas that were meant to be involved in intimacy are now associated with pain and have been poked and prodded by people other than intimate partners. Many patients tell me, "I have been through so much, I have no privacy left." Those body parts now become associated with negative feelings versus only warm, positive ones. That is something well worth communicating to partners, so they can understand any resistance you might present, and that way, feelings don't get hurt unnecessarily when you "aren't in the mood." There are specially trained psychologists who can help with counseling and reaffirmation of your sexuality. Ask your health care providers to supply a referral. Support groups may also provide a way to gather information on sensitive issues (see end of Chapter 11). Please don't stay silent; if you don't talk about your issues and concerns, they will not get resolved.

Women

Women consistently rate their IBD symptoms at higher levels of severity than men. Both men and women are concerned with attractiveness, intimacy, and sexual performance, but women tend to have stronger concerns about self-image and feeling alone and are more fearful of having children.[294] Active disease can lead to fatigue and loss of libido, in addition to the embarrassment of fecal incontinence; these are just more good reasons to work to keep your disease in remission. Of all the medications we use to do this, steroids are the type linked to weight gain, acne, and mood swings, all of which contribute to poor self-image.

Crohn's disease that involves the rectal and vaginal areas can be physically deforming, as well as cause painful intercourse and self-consciousness. The presence of an ostomy or other surgical scars can also lead to lower self-esteem. It is difficult to feel sexy or to enjoy sex if you are not comfortable with who you are and how your body looks and functions.

So, what can you do? Let's start with the physical first. I counsel women with Crohn's disease to avoid thong underwear and bikinis. The band can be particularly irritating to the anal canal and can cause further irritation to skin tags, fissures, or fistulas that are present.

Women with a stoma often have self-image issues and serious concerns about attracting a partner. What I recommend for women in this situation is wearing crotchless underwear and teddies, or teddies with snap crotches, so that the abdominal wall is covered and the groin area is exposed, which is the opposite of most underwear.

Men

Men tend to be most concerned about performance issues. It's reassuring that erectile dysfunction does not appear to be any more of a risk than for men without IBD.[295] Active inflammation of IBD rarely causes erectile problems. One of the causes of erectile dysfunction is undiagnosed or untreated depression. Watch for signs of depression in yourself and get the help you need.

Loss of libido can certainly result from the discomfort and symptoms of active disease, but it can also be caused by a decreased testosterone level. Testosterone is a sex hormone made from cholesterol. If there is not enough cholesterol in the body because of diarrhea or poor absorption in the bowel, then the body cannot produce enough testosterone. The solution comes through improving nutrition and supplementing the testosterone level, for example, by wearing a testosterone patch.

One of the risks of the J pouch procedure is the possibility of retrograde ejaculation following surgery, but as surgeons gain more experience with this procedure, this complication appears to happen less and less.

Men are also concerned about their ability to father children—and about the likelihood of passing along IBD to the child. Preliminary genetic studies have suggested that the risk of passing along IBD is stronger from the mother than the father, but that has not been proven conclusively. Overall, there is no difference in sperm health in males with IBD than in men without. A few years ago, there was a very controversial study that suggested men on 6-mercaptopurine (6-MP) had an increased risk of fathering a child with a birth complication or birth defect.[296] The study was small and has not been reproduced by other investigators. In fact, there have been two other larger studies that refute any differences in sperm quality, number, or motility between men on 6-MP and those not on 6-MP.[297–299] It is important to remember that sulfasalazine does cause a significantly lower sperm count, which is reversed when you stop taking the drug. The sperm-lowering effect is not dose dependent, which means it would happen even on just one tablet a day.

The Menstrual Cycle

Girls diagnosed with IBD before or during puberty may have a delay in when they get their first period (called *menarche*). This can be caused by chronic inflammation or poor nutrition that directly affects the body's ability to produce the necessary sex hormones. Chronic inflammation can shut down the normal hormonal signals that the body uses to "talk" to itself. This leads to decreased levels of hormones in women that can result in irregular or absent periods, and men can have decreased sex drive from too little testosterone. Menarche usually occurs once active disease is treated appropriately.

Disease activity can also affect the menstrual cycle and result in irregular or skipped periods or an increase in disease symptoms before or during the time of menstruation. A study in which I participated confirmed that patients with IBD had more GI-related symptoms during periods than the general population.[300] These symptoms occurred in a predictable fashion at the same time every month and included diarrhea, abdominal pain similar to their disease, and constipation. A lot of women appear to experience worse symptoms either right before or during their periods, and some consider these to be "miniflares." In reality, this is a milder and predictable phenomenon. Be conservative in treating these symptoms because they tend to go away a few days after the period. Also, be careful of over-the-counter medications for menstrual symptoms such as Pamprin and Midol. Those that contain high quantities of naproxen or aspirin can cause additional inflammation (see Chapter 6) and damage to the lining of the GI tract. I counsel my patients not to use these medications unless absolutely necessary because of the risk of a disease flare.

Stacey had fairly well controlled ulcerative colitis, but definitely noticed that her "PMS" included more abdominal cramps and looser stools than the rest of the month. She wasn't sure if these were flares of her disease or not. She finally asked me if it was normal to have more stools before her period—almost like a "mini-flare" every month. I had her track her symptoms through two full cycles, and we reviewed what she had recorded. The pattern was that during the week before her period was due, she had more GI symptoms, which went away the following week. In the past, she had been given steroids to treat her symptoms but didn't like the way the steroids made her feel. Instead, I recommended that she increase the amount of her 5-ASA by 1.2 g the week before the PMS to help prevent the symptoms. She did this and noticed a difference the next month. Now she takes a higher dose to prevent these symptoms and during the rest of the month takes her normal maintenance dose.

Some women have such debilitating GI symptoms related to menstruation that stopping it altogether is the only way to provide relief. This can be achieved with short-term injectable contraceptives (Depo-Provera) or hormones (Lupron). Although your IBD symptoms do not make a hysterectomy medically necessary, women who have a hysterectomy for gynecologic or other reasons find their IBD symptoms improve.

Menopause

Menopause, whether it occurs naturally or is brought on by surgery to remove the uterus, leads to many changes in a woman's body. Just as oral contraceptives and pregnancy can help control symptoms of IBD, research suggests that some of the gastrointestinal symptoms associated with IBD decrease in women who have experienced menopause.

Women with ulcerative colitis are no more likely to enter menopause early than women without IBD. There are some data, however, to suggest that women with Crohn's disease may enter menopause earlier than otherwise healthy women, but we have yet to discover why this is so.[301]

A recent study done by my colleagues and I revealed that post-menopausal women with IBD are just as likely to have a flare as women that are premenopausal.[302] This study demonstrated that hormone replacement therapy (HRT) had a protective effect on IBD disease activity and that this effect appears to be dose dependent. This means the higher the HRT dose, the less likely a flare. More research on the relationship between exogenous hormones and IBD needs to be done before HRT can be recommended for all women with IBD undergoing menopause. We will continue to conduct research and share findings in an ongoing effort to improve the health and quality of life of all people with IBD.

Pap Smears

Women taking immunosuppressant drugs, such as steroids and azathioprine or 6-MP, long term are more likely to have abnormalities of the cervix found by Pap smear compared with the general rate or women using biologic therapies.[303, 304] When found, these abnormalities tend to be the more serious type. This is probably related to the reduced ability to clear any human papilloma virus (HPV) infection. Women with IBD who take immunomodulators are considered at high risk and need annual Pap smears with timely follow up of any abnormal results. Girls and young women with IBD should consider having the HPV vaccine, which is recommended for those between the ages of 9 and 26. It is unclear at this time whether women older than 26 would receive benefit, and trials are underway to study this question.

Contraception

Contraception in women with IBD who do not wish to become pregnant differs only slightly from that for healthy women. The most important goal remains the selection of the most reliable method of birth control.

- Barrier methods such as a condom or diaphragm are acceptable but not quite as effective as other choices, such as birth control pills.
- Intrauterine devices (IUDs) are not usually recommended, because abdominal pain from IBD could be mistaken for pelvic inflammatory disease. Irritation or infection that is sometimes caused by the IUD can be mistaken for active IBD, which would delay getting the correct treatment.
- Oral contraceptives or birth control pills (OCs) present some challenges for women with IBD. Most OCs are absorbed from the small bowel, and this absorption is key for the contraceptive's effectiveness. If it takes too long to pass through the bowel, if you have an ileostomy (there may not be an adequate length of bowel to allow for absorption), or if there is impaired absorption because of inflammation, the contraceptive can fail. Many antibiotics carry a warning of decreased effectiveness of OCs when the two are taken in combination, but in speaking with experts in the field, I could not find anyone who really finds this to be true. It may be a theoretical outcome based on what happens in a test tube.

The data regarding the safety of OCs in IBD are conflicting.[305] Preliminary studies suggest that taking OCs increases the risk for developing Crohn's disease and ulcerative colitis, but this did not take into account tobacco use, which is a risk factor just on its own. Reports from Europe, where birth control pills contain a higher amount of estrogen, continue to show modest increases in the risk of developing Crohn's disease, after adjusting for cigarette use. However, I performed two case-controlled studies (in the United States) that showed no increased risk of either ulcerative colitis or Crohn's disease from OC use.

Other data suggest that OC use may make IBD worse. Two small studies where patients were followed over a long period found that those taking OCs had an increased risk of flares in their Crohn's disease after it had gone into remission. No information is available for a possible similar risk in ulcerative colitis.

There are no standard guidelines for OC use, in part because there are so many types available (more than 70!), so this is an individual decision. The variable amounts of progesterone and estrogen determine the side effects. In discussing whether to use an OC, and which one, with your health care provider, consider your overall health, any previous pregnancies, and your personal preferences. It is best to try a pill that contains the lowest amount of estrogen possible to lower the risk of blood clots. Because people with Crohn's disease also have a tendency to develop blood clots, it is especially risky to take OCs and smoke—so don't smoke.

Fertility

Up to 7% of couples in America are infertile. Do not be too quick to blame your IBD if you are trying unsuccessfully to have a baby. However, in some circumstances, fertility in an IBD patient is definitely decreased.

- Men who take sulfasalazine tend to have a decreased sperm count, but this is totally reversible when you stop taking the drug.
- Women who have active inflammation may have irregular periods, which decrease the chances of getting pregnant.
- Women with active disease may have scarring of their fallopian tubes, making it difficult for an egg to travel from the ovary to the uterus for fertilization.
- Women who have had a J pouch procedure for colitis are significantly less able to get pregnant than women with ulcerative colitis who have not had the operation, which is the same as in the general population. The construction of the pouch, which sits deep in the pelvis, creates scar tissue that we believe prevents eggs from traveling from the ovary to the uterus. Fewer eggs end up in the uterus for possible fertilization. The risk of infertility in someone with a J pouch is about 50% to

60%. Having the procedure laparoscopically does not improve this rate.

Women with ulcerative colitis facing surgery but concerned about future fertility have several options. The first is to have just the first stage of the surgery and a temporary stoma until your childbearing is done. The colon is removed but without manipulation in the pelvis to cause scarring. However, if you have not yet met the potential father of your children, you may not want to have a stoma. Another option is an operation to attach the small intestine to the rectum. While this protects fertility and does not require a stoma, there is still some disease in place in the rectum. Because the purpose of the operation is to remove the disease and restore health, when an actively diseased rectum is left in place, you may not feel any better after the operation. This can cause psychological problems like depression as well as physical problems. In addition, without a colon, the number of bowel movements increases significantly, which can really diminish your sense of well-being. Having a J pouch does not mean that you will be infertile; but reduced fertility due to the scarring is a fact that you'll need to keep in mind when weighing medical versus surgical treatments. Women with J pouches do not appear to have less success using artificial means of becoming pregnant if necessary.

Women with Crohn's disease have slightly lower rates of fertility compared with the general population, probably because of the effect of inflammation in the pelvis. This can cause scarring of the fallopian tubes and problems with proper ovulation by the ovaries. Women with Crohn's disease are also more likely to suffer irregular periods and malnutrition.

Pregnancy

Having a baby is exciting but also quite stressful. Getting pregnant, staying pregnant, delivering, and then caring for your newborn can all affect your overall health. Most women with IBD are in their child-bearing years, and the thought of pregnancy can be quite overwhelming. I want to reassure you that, for most women with IBD, pregnancy is not dangerous, as some may make it out to be. The medications we use now allow patients to be healthier and disease free for longer intervals than in the past—so contraception may be more of an issue.

Plan Your Pregnancy

Be as proactive as you can about the timing of conception; the healthier you are at the time of conception, no matter what your underlying condition may be, the better chance of a successful pregnancy. Discuss with your health care provider the medications you are taking and whether any changes or accommodations need to be made if you get pregnant. For example, if you have reflux disease and take a proton pump inhibitor, this class of medications is considered pretty safe during pregnancy. In fact, your reflux may get worse during pregnancy, so it is important to stay on your medications.

During pregnancy, you need to be carefully monitored by both your gastroenterology health care provider and your obstetrician for signs of active disease and fetal complications. Pick an obstetrician before you get pregnant, if possible. Let him or her know your medical history so that medications can be discussed ahead of time. Some obstetricians have strong feelings about certain medications, and an open discussion will help avoid problems once you are pregnant. And finally, find out about the gastrointestinal symptoms that are part of normal pregnancy. These include constipation and reflux, especially as you enter the third trimester.

How Pregnancy Affects IBD

If you are in remission at the time of conception, getting pregnant does not increase the risk of a flare.[306] The risk of a flare over a 9-month period is not zero, but being pregnant will not increase this chance. If, however, you have active disease at the time of conception, then we talk about the "rule of thirds." One third of women will get better, one third will stay the same, and one third will get worse. I have had several women tell me their disease was never under such good control as when they were pregnant. When they flare, they contemplate getting pregnant to control the disease. (I do not necessarily support that idea!)

We think the reason for the rule-of-thirds phenomenon has to do with the amount of genetic material shared between the mother and the fetus.[307] The more DNA that came from the father, the more "foreign" the fetus is to the mother. In order to not "reject" this foreign entity growing inside her, her body downregulates her own immune system. In the process, her autoimmune disease goes into remission. We believe that those women who go into remission are carrying babies that have more paternal DNA than maternal. The more maternal DNA that matches the baby, the worse her disease will do. Again, this only applies to women whose disease is active at the time of conception.

How IBD Affects Pregnancy

Your disease activity at the time of conception is the strongest predictor of your pregnancy outcome. Having active IBD during conception is associated with a higher rate of spontaneous abortion. Having active IBD during the course of pregnancy increases the rate of premature birth and the chance for a small-for-gestational-age, low-birth-weight infant.[308]

But regardless of disease activity, women with either ulcerative colitis or Crohn's disease have higher rates of premature births. Women with Crohn's disease have an increased risk for low-birth-weight and small-for-gestational-age infants. It is not clear why this is, and it seems to occur in women with both inactive and active disease. It may have to do with nutritional factors preconception and at conception time and the fact that more women with Crohn's smoke (even during pregnancy) and are more prone to anemia.

Despite some of these sobering statements, most babies are normal and healthy. Their APGAR scores are in the normal range, and there does not appear to be any increased risk for birth defects in children born to mothers with IBD.

FAQs

Which medications are safe for me to use? In general, most medications that we use to treat IBD are considered low risk for pregnancy. There is some disagreement regarding the immunomodulators and biologics, but most agree that patients require some type of continued treatment through a pregnancy to keep disease activity under control.

- Methotrexate, thalidomide, and diphenoxylate (Lomotil) should be stopped before a planned pregnancy or as soon as pregnancy is diagnosed.
- Metronidazole appears to be low risk and can be used for longer periods of time than previously thought safe.
- Ciprofloxacin is not to be taken during pregnancy because of its potential effect on the cartilage of a growing fetus. For IBD purposes, we try to minimize the use of antibiotics.
- Mesalamine agents are safe in pregnancy. If you take sulfa-salazine, you also need to take folic acid (2 mg daily). This is more than what comes in a normal prenatal vitamin.
- Prednisone is considered low risk during pregnancy if you need it to control IBD. There is an increased risk of gestational diabetes and large-birth-weight babies. Cleft palate has been associated with steroid using during pregnancy, but this appears to be the case in asthmatic mothers and not ones with IBD.
- The use of azathioprine and 6-MP is controversial. Most data in IBD support their safety in pregnancy.[295] We need to balance the risk to the mother of flaring against the theoretical risk of increased birth defects in the fetus. If you have had disease that is difficult to treat and is now in remission with this agent, I recommend that you continue to manage your IBD with 6-MP or azathioprine throughout the pregnancy. The thing to keep in mind is that if you really want to be off these drugs during pregnancy, you should stop taking them at least 3 months before trying to conceive. The drugs take a while to completely leave your system. If you are taking them and think you might be pregnant,

do a pregnancy test immediately. The first 6 to 8 weeks of pregnancy are when all of the fetal organs develop, and if you are already that far along in the pregnancy, stopping your therapy just puts your disease at risk and does not prevent the fetal exposure. Another point is that these medications were first developed in the 1950s to treat leukemia and the doses used to treat leukemia were much higher than those used to treat IBD. The birth defects seen with azathioprine and 6-MP were first reported with the higher doses. At lower doses, the risk does not appear to be anywhere near what it is at higher doses. The decision to continue or stop these medications during pregnancy is an individual one, and no one-size-fits-all approach is appropriate here.

■ Cyclosporine, when needed, is safer than surgery for a pregnant ulcerative colitis patient with severe disease that is not responding to intravenous steroids. Fortunately, the need to use this drug is rare.

■ The safety of the biologics is still an ongoing investigation. Remicade has been used the most to date, with no apparent increased risk to the fetus or the mother. In fact, we have even initiated Remicade during pregnancy to control disease, with no increase in birth defects.[309] We do not have as much data for the newer biologics, but it is logical to assume that they would not increase the rate of birth defects either. We have been able to measure Remicade in the blood of newborns so we know that it crosses the placenta, but it is metabolized over time and does not appear to cause any effects to the immune system of the infant.[310] Because we know that the biologics cross the placenta, we have women stop receiving this therapy in the third trimester because this is the time that the largest amount of medicine will cross the placenta. The best case is to minimize the amount that the fetus gets exposed to while treating the mother. For women on Remicade, we recommend that the dose not be increased as your weight increases during pregnancy. The other IBD medications are not weight-based for dosing, so you would continue the same doses.

What are the chances my child will get IBD? As discussed in Chapter 1, the risk of a child getting IBD from a single parent is low, between 3% and 7%.[8] If both parents have IBD, then the chance increases to almost 50%. However, it is not 100%, which indicates that it takes more than genetic factors to cause this disease.

What is the effect of smoking? As you might expect, smoking has been shown to increase the likelihood of having a relapse of your IBD and it decreases your response to medications for Crohn's disease. For the baby's health and your own, please stop smoking before and during pregnancy.

Do I have to have a cesarean section? In general, women with IBD can have a normal vaginal delivery unless, for obstetric or personal reasons, a C-section is recommended. If you have active perianal disease at delivery time, having a C-section avoids making this condition worse due to the trauma of the birthing process. If you have a J pouch, a vaginal delivery won't harm the pouch. However, some surgeons recommend that you have a C-section anyway, because retaining proper anal sphincter function is critical. Having a vaginal delivery can compromise the function of the anal sphincter, with or without a pouch. This can happen immediately from the trauma of the pushing during delivery, or it can be delayed and happen because of the experience but appear sometime in the future. This can take decades to occur, like the aging process that causes "sagging" of the muscles in the pelvic floor that leads to common problems with incontinence of stool or urine.

What if I need an endoscopy? There is no need for routine procedures during pregnancy, but if one is required to assess disease activity or obtain tissue samples, then a flexible sigmoidoscopy is usually adequate. Rarely do you need a full colonoscopy. Flexible sigmoidoscopies can be performed with a tap water enema preparation and little or no sedation. There is no evidence to suggest that undergoing a flexible sigmoidoscopy increases the risk for premature rupture of membranes, contractions, or other problems with the pregnancy.[311]

Can I nurse? This is a personal decision and should not be forced on you. You must decide whether you want to nurse your baby and then factor in your medications, because having to stop taking them may make your condition worse.

- Breastfeeding is not recommended when you are on antibiotics.
- Breastfeeding is allowed when you are using steroids.
- Breastfeeding is not allowed if you are taking cyclosporine.
- Breastfeeding is allowed when you are on 5-ASA products.
- Breastfeeding is not encouraged when you are on azathioprine or 6-MP based on old information. Newer information suggests that the benefits of breastfeeding outweigh the miniscule exposure that the infant gets to drugs found in the breast milk.[312] A reasonable compromise, knowing that drug levels are highest in the first milk of the morning, is to take your medication at night and then "pump and dump" the first milk of the morning. Feed the baby a bottle at that first feeding and then nurse the remainder of the day.
- Breastfeeding is not currently recommended for mothers taking a biologic, but this is based on the lack of adequate data regarding levels of the medicine in breast milk. There have now been reports of several patients taking Remicade while nursing, and no Remicade has been found in the breast milk.[313] It is assumed that the other biologic agents are also not actively secreted into mother's milk. Even if there is some level of the drug in the milk, it is a protein that the baby's body would break down with stomach acid. Therefore, I allow my patients on these agents to nurse.

A final note for nursing mothers, I do not recommend the use of the herbal supplement fennugreek to try to enhance milk production. Some lactation consultants recommend it, but it can cause rectal bleeding, which is obviously a bad thing for those with Crohn's disease or ulcerative colitis.

References

1. Loftus CG, Loftus EV Jr, Harmsen WS, et al. Update on the incidence and prevalence of Crohn's disease and ulcerative colitis in Olmsted County, Minnesota, 1940–2000. *Inflamm Bowel Dis* 2007;13(3): 254–61.

2. Sands BE, Grabert S. Epidemiology of inflammatory bowel disease and overview of pathogenesis. *Med Health R I* 2009;92(3):73–77.

3. Koloski NA, Bret L, Radford-Smith G. Hygiene hypothesis in inflammatory bowel disease: a critical review of the literature. *World J Gastroenterol* 2008;14(2):165–73.

4. Burgmann T, Clara I, Graff L, et al. The Manitoba Inflammatory Bowel Disease Cohort Study: prolonged symptoms before diagnosis—how much is irritable bowel syndrome? *Clin Gastroenterol Hepatol* 2006;4(5): 614–20.

5. Halder SL, Locke GR 3rd, Schleck CD, et al. Natural history of functional gastrointestinal disorders: a 12-year longitudinal population-based study. *Gastroenterology* 2007;133(3):799–807.

6. Astegiano M, Pellicano R, Sguazzini C, et al. Clinical approach to irritable bowel syndrome. *Minerva Gastroenterol Dietol* 2008;54(3): 251–57.

7. Simrén M, Axelsson J, Gillberg R, et al. Quality of life in inflammatory bowel disease in remission: the impact of IBS-like symptoms and associated psychological factors. *Am J Gastroenterol* 2002;97(2): 389–96.

8. Cho JH. The genetics and immunopathogenesis of inflammatory bowel disease. *Nat Rev Immunol* 2008;8(6):458–66.

9. Noomen CG, Hommes DW, Fidder HH. Update on genetics in inflammatory disease. *Best Pract Res Clin Gastroenterol* 2009;23(2):233–43.

10. Hisamatsu T, Ogata H, Hibi T. Innate immunity in inflammatory bowel disease: state of the art. *Curr Opin Gastroenterol* 2008;24(4): 448–54.

11. Slonim AE, Bulone L, Damore MB, et al. A preliminary study of growth hormone therapy for Crohn's disease. *N Engl J Med* 2000;342(22): 1633–37.

12. Oyama Y, Craig RM, Traynor AE, et al. Autologous hematopoietic stem cell transplantation in patients with refractory Crohn's disease. *Gastroenterology* 2005;128(3):552–63.

13. Van der Heide F, Dijkstra A, Weersma RK, et al. Effects of active and passive smoking on disease course of Crohn's disease and ulcerative colitis. *Inflamm Bowel Dis* 2009;15(8):1199–207.

14. Mendoza JL, Lana R, Díaz-Rubio M. Mycobacterium avium subspecies paratuberculosis and its relationship with Crohn's disease. *World J Gastroenterol* 2009;15(4):417–22.

15. Selby W, Pavli P, Crotty B, et al., Antibiotics in Crohn's Disease Study Group. Two-year combination antibiotic therapy with clarithromycin,

rifabutin, and clofazimine for Crohn's disease. *Gastroenterology* 2007; 132(7):2313–39.

16. Sainsbury A, Heatley RV. Psychosocial factors in the quality of life of patients with inflammatory bowel disease (review). *Aliment Pharmacol Ther* 2005;21(5):499–508.

17. Walker JR, Ediger JP, Graff LA, et al. The Manitoba IBD Cohort Study: a population-based study of the prevalence of lifetime and 12-month anxiety and mood disorders. *Am J Gastroenterol* 2008; 103(8):1989–97.

18. Kübler-Ross E, Wessler S, Avioli LV. On death and dying. *JAMA* 1972; 221(2):174–79.

19. Tooson JD, Gates LK Jr. Bowel preparation before colonoscopy: choosing the best lavage regimen. *Postgrad Med* 1996;100(2):203–204, 207–12, 214.

20. Rubin DT, Siegel CA, Kane SV, et al. Impact of ulcerative colitis from patients' and physicians' perspectives: results from the UC: NORMAL survey. *Inflamm Bowel Dis* 2009;15(4):581–88.

21. Lewis JD, Aberra FN, Lichtenstein GR, et al. Seasonal variation in flares of inflammatory bowel disease. *Gastroenterology* 2004;126(3): 665–73.

22. Karban A, Eliakim R. Effect of smoking on inflammatory bowel disease: is it disease or organ specific? *World J Gastroenterol* 2007;13(15): 2150–52.

23. Singh S, Graff LA, Bernstein CN. Do NSAIDs, antibiotics, infections, or stress trigger flares in IBD? *Am J Gastroenterol* 2009;104(5): 1298–313.

24. Reddy D, Siegel CA, Sands BE, Kane S. Possible association between isotretinoin and inflammatory bowel disease. *Am J Gastroenterol* 2006; 101(7):1569–73.

25. Cosnes J, Cattan S, Blain A, et al. Long-term evolution of disease behavior of Crohn's disease. *Inflamm Bowel Dis* 2002;8(4):244–50.

26. Devlin SM, Dubinsky MC. Determination of serologic and genetic markers aid in the determination of the clinical course and severity of patients with IBD. *Inflamm Bowel Dis* 2008;14(1):125–28.

27. Sipponen T, Kärkkäinen P, Savilahti E, et al. Correlation of faecal calprotectin and lactoferrin with an endoscopic score for Crohn's disease and histological findings. *Aliment Pharmacol Ther* 2008;28(10): 1221–29.

28. Gisbert JP, McNicholl AG, Gomollon F. Questions and answers on the role of fecal lactoferrin as a biological marker in inflammatory bowel disease. *Inflamm Bowel Dis* 2009;15(11):1746–54.

29. Solem CA, Loftus EV Jr, Fletcher JG, et al. Small-bowel imaging in Crohn's disease: a prospective, blinded, 4-way comparison trial. *Gastrointest Endosc* 2008;68(2):255–66.

30. Melmed GY, Elashoff R, Chen GC, et al. Predicting a change in diagnosis from ulcerative colitis to Crohn's disease: a nested, case-control study. *Clin Gastroenterol Hepatol* 2007;5(5):602–608.

31. Tangri V, Chande N. Microscopic colitis: an update. *J Clin Gastroenterol* 2009;43(4):293–96.

32. Chande N, McDonald JW, Macdonald JK. Interventions for treating collagenous colitis. *Cochrane Database Syst Rev* 2008; Apr 16(2):CD003575.

33. Dick AP, Grayson MJ, Carpenter RG, Petrie A. Controlled trial of sulphasalazine in the treatment of ulcerative colitis. *Gut* 1964;50:437–42.

34. Dew, MJ, Hughes, P, Harries, AD, et al. Maintenance of remission in ulcerative colitis with oral preparation of 5-aminosalicylic acid. *Br Med J (Clin Res Ed)* 1982;285(6347):1012.

35. Schroeder KW, Tremaine WJ, Ilstrup DM. Coated oral 5-aminosalicylic acid therapy for mildly to moderately active ulcerative colitis: a randomized study. *N Engl J Med* 1987;317(26):1625–29.

36. Mulder CJ, Tytgat GN, Weterman IT, et al. Double-blind comparison of slow-release 5-aminosalicylate and sulfasalazine in remission maintenance in ulcerative colitis. *Gastroenterology* 1988;95(6):1449–53.

37. Riley, SA, Mani, V, Goodman, MJ, et al. Comparison of delayed release 5-aminosalicylic acid (mesalazine) and sulphasalazine in the treatment of mild to moderate ulcerative colitis relapse. *Gut* 1988;29(5):669–74.

38. Zinberg J, Molinas S, Das KM. Double-blind placebo-controlled study of olsalazine in the treatment of ulcerative colitis. *Am J Gastroenterol* 1990;85(5):562–66.

39. Levine DS, Riff DS, Pruitt R, et al. A randomized, double blind, dose-response comparison of balsalazide (6.75 g), balsalazide (2.25 g), and mesalamine (2.4 g) in the treatment of active, mild-to-moderate ulcerative colitis. *Am J Gastroenterol* 2002;97(6):1398–407.

40. Hanauer SB, Sandborn WJ, Kornbluth A, et al. Delayed-release oral mesalamine at 4.8 g/day (800 mg tablet) for the treatment of moderately active ulcerative colitis: the ASCEND II Trial. *Am J Gastroenterol* 2005; 100(11):2478–85.

41. Kamm MA, Sandborn WJ, Gassull M, et al. Once-daily, high-concentration MMX mesalamine in active ulcerative colitis. *Gastroenterology* 2000;132(1):66–75.

42. Sandborn WJ, Kamm MA, Lichtenstein GR, et al. MMX Multi Matrix System mesalazine for the induction of remission in patients with mild-to-moderate ulcerative colitis: a combined analysis of two randomized, double-blind, placebo-controlled trials. *Aliment Pharmacol Ther* 2007; 26(2):205–15.

43. Scherl EJ, Pruitt R, Gordon GL, et al. Safety and efficacy of a new 3.3 g b.i.d. tablet formulation in patients with mild-to-moderately-active ulcerative colitis: a multicenter, randomized, double-blind, placebo-controlled study. *Am J Gastroenterol* 2009;104(6):1452–59.

44. Summers, RW, Switz, DM, Sessions, JT, et al. National Cooperative Crohn's disease study: results of drug treatment. *Gastroenterology* 1979; 77(4 Pt. 2):847–69.

45. Hanauer SB, Stromberg U. Oral Pentasa in the treatment of active Crohn's disease: a meta-analysis of double-blind, placebo-controlled trials. *Clin Gastroenterol Hepatol* 2004;2(5):379–88.

46. Velayos FS, Terdiman JP, Walsh JM. Effect of 5-aminosalicylate use on colorectal cancer and dysplasia risk: a systematic review and meta-analysis of observational studies. *Am J Gastroenterol* 2005;100(6): 1345–53.

47. Safdi M, DeMicco M, Sninsky C, et al. A double-blind comparison of oral versus rectal mesalamine versus combination therapy in the treatment of distal ulcerative colitis. *Am J Gastroenterol* 1997;92(10): 1867–71.

48. Marteau P, Probert CS, Lindgren S, et al. Combined oral and enema treatment with Pentasa (mesalazine) is superior to oral therapy alone in patients with extensive mild/moderate active ulcerative colitis: a randomised, double blind, placebo controlled study. *Gut* 2005;54(7): 960–65.

49. Dignass AU, Bokemeyer B, Adamek H, et al. Mesalamine once daily is more effective than twice daily in patients with quiescent ulcerative colitis. *Clin Gastroenterol Hepatol* 2009;7(7):762–69.

50. Loftus EV Jr, Kane SV, Bjorkman D. Systematic review: short-term adverse effects of 5-aminosalicylic acid agents in the treatment of ulcerative colitis. *Aliment Pharmacol Ther* 2004;19(2):179–89.

51. Brandt LJ, Bernstein LH, Boley SJ, Frank MS. Metronidazole therapy for perineal Crohn's disease: a follow-up study. *Gastroenterology* 1982; 83(2):383–87.

52. Colombel JF, Lemann M, Cassagnou M, et al., Groupe d'Etudes Therapeutiques des Affections Inflammatoires Digestives (GETAID). A controlled trial comparing ciprofloxacin with mesalazine for the treatment of active Crohn's disease. *Am J Gastroenterol* 1999;94(3):674–78.

53. Issa M, Vijayapal A, Graham MB, et al. Impact of Clostridium difficile on inflammatory bowel disease. *Clin Gastroenterol Hepatol* 2007;5(3): 345–51.

54. Steinhart AH, Ewe K, Griffiths AM, et al. Corticosteroids for maintenance of remission in Crohn's disease. *Cochrane Database Syst Rev* 2003; (4):CD000301.

55. Bossa F, Fiorella S, Caruso N, et al. Continuous infusion versus bolus administration of steroids in severe attacks of ulcerative colitis: a randomized, double-blind trial. *Am J Gastroenterol* 2007;102(3):601–608.

56. Turner D, Walsh CM, Steinhart AH, Griffiths AM. Response to corticosteroids in severe ulcerative colitis: a systematic review of the literature and a meta-regression. *Clin Gastroenterol Hepatol* 2007;5(1): 103–10.

57. Marshall JK, Irvine JK. Rectal aminosalicylate therapy in distal ulcerative colitis: a meta-analysis. *Aliment Pharmacol Ther* 1995;9(3): 293–300.

58. Marshall JK, Irvine EJ. Rectal corticosteroids versus alternative treatments in ulcerative colitis: a meta-analysis. *Gut* 1997;40(6):775–81.

59. Hanauer S, Good LI, Goodman MW. Long-term use of mesalamine (Rowasa) suppositories in remission maintenance of ulcerative proctitis. *Am J Gastroenterol* 2000;95(7):1749–54.

60. Lichtenstein GR, Feagan BG, Cohen RD, et al. Serious infections and mortality in association with therapies for Crohn's disease: TREAT registry. *Clin Gastroenterol Hepatol* 2006;4(5):621–30. Erratum: *Clin Gastroenterol Hepatol* 2006;4(7):931.

61. Thomsen OO, Cortot A, Jewell D, et al., International Budesonide-Mesalamine Study Group. A comparison of budesonide and mesalamine for active Crohn's disease. *N Engl J Med* 1998;339(6):370–74. Erratum: *N Engl J Med* 2001;345(22):1652.

62. Benchimol EI, Seow CH, Otley AR, Steinhart AH. Budesonide for maintenance of remission in Crohn's disease (Review). *Cochrane Database Syst Rev* 2009;Jan 21(1):CD002913.

63. Tremaine WJ, Hanauer SB, Katz S, et al., Budesonide CIR United States Study Group. Budesonide CIR capsules (once or twice daily divided-dose) in active Crohn's disease: a randomized placebo-controlled study in the United States. *Am J Gastroenterol* 2002;97(7):1748–54.

64. Gross V, Bar-Meir S, Lavy A, et al., International Budesonide Foam Study Group. Budesonide foam versus budesonide enema in active

ulcerative proctitis and proctosigmoiditis. *Aliment Pharmacol Ther* 2006; 23(2):303–12.

65. Seow CH, Benchimol EI, Griffiths AM, et al. Budesonide for induction of remission in Crohn's disease (Review). *Cochrane Database Syst Rev* 2008;Jul 16(3):CD000296.

66. Tursi A, Giorgetti GM, Brandimarte G, Elisei W. Safety and effectiveness of long-term budesonide treatment in maintaining remission in patients with mild-to-moderate Crohn's disease. *Inflamm Bowel Dis* 2007;13(9):1184–86.

67. Lindgren S, Löfberg R, Bergholm L, Hellblom M, Carling L, Ung KA, Schiöler R, Unge P, Wallin C, Ström M, Persson T, Suhr OB. Effect of budesonide enema on remission and relapse rate in distal ulcerative colitis and proctitis. *Scand J Gastroenterol* 2002;37(6):705–10.

68. Korelitz BI, Present DH. Favorable effect of 6-mercaptopurine on fistulae of Crohn's disease. *Dig Dis Sci* 1985;30(1):58–64.

69. Present DH, Korelitz BI, Wisch N, et al. Treatment of Crohn's disease with 6-mercaptopurine: a long-term, randomized, double-blind study. *N Engl J Med* 1980;302(18):981–87.

70. Cassinotti A, Actis GC, Duca P, et al. Maintenance treatment with azathioprine in ulcerative colitis: outcome and predictive factors after drug withdrawal. *Am J Gastroenterol* 2009;104(11):2760–67.

71. Mantzaris GJ, Sfakianakis M, Archavlis E, et al. A prospective randomized observer-blind 2-year trial of azathioprine monotherapy versus azathioprine and olsalazine for the maintenance of remission of steroid-dependent ulcerative colitis. *Am J Gastroenterol* 2004;99(6): 1122–28.

72. Gisbert JP, Linares PM, McNicholl AG, et al. Meta-analysis: the efficacy of azathioprine and mercaptopurine in ulcerative colitis. *Aliment Pharmacol Ther* 2009;30(2):126–37.

73. Kandiel A, Fraser AG, Korelitz BI, et al. Increased risk of lymphoma among inflammatory bowel disease patients treated with azathioprine and 6-mercaptopurine. *Gut* 2005;54(8):1121–25.

74. Dayharsh GA, Loftus EV Jr, Sandborn WJ, et al. Epstein-Barr virus-positive lymphoma in patients with inflammatory bowel disease treated with azathioprine or 6-mercaptopurine. *Gastroenterology* 2002;122(1): 72–77.

75. Feagan BG, Fedorak RN, Irvine EJ, et al., North American Crohn's Study Group Investigators. A comparison of methotrexate with placebo for the maintenance of remission in Crohn's disease. *N Engl J Med* 2000; 342(22):1627–32.

76. Oren R, Arber N, Odes S, et al. Methotrexate in chronic active ulcerative colitis: a double-blind, randomized, Israeli multicenter trial. *Gastroenterology* 1996;110(5):1416–21.

77. Mate-Jimenez J, Hermida C, Cantero-Perona J, Moreno-Otero R. 6-Mercaptopurine or methotrexate added to prednisone induces and maintains remission in steroid-dependent inflammatory bowel disease. *Eur J Gastroenterol Hepatol* 2000;12(11):1227–33.

78. Kozarek RA, Patterson DJ, Gelfand MD, et al. Methotrexate induces clinical and histologic remission in patients with refractory inflammatory bowel disease. *Ann Intern Med* 1989;110(5):353–56.

79. Baron TH, Truss CD, Elson CO. Low-dose oral methotrexate in refractory inflammatory bowel disease. *Dig Dis Sci* 1993;38(10):1851–56.

80. Chande N, MacDonald JK, McDonald JW. Methotrexate for induction of remission in ulcerative colitis. *Cochrane Database Syst Rev* 2007;(4): CD006618.

81. Te HS, Schiano TD, Kuan SF, et al. Hepatic effects of long-term methotrexate use in the treatment of inflammatory bowel disease. *Am J Gastroenterol* 2000;95(11):3150–56.

82. Lichtiger S, Present DH, Kornbluth A, et al. Cyclosporine in severe ulcerative colitis refractory to steroid therapy. *N Engl J Med* 1994; 330(26):1841–45.

83. Actis GC, Ottobrelli A, Pera A, et al. Continuously infused cyclosporine at low dose is sufficient to avoid emergency colectomy in acute attacks of ulcerative colitis. *J Clin Gastroenterol* 1993;17(1):10–13.

84. Cohen RD, Stein R, Hanauer SB. Intravenous cyclosporine in ulcerative colitis: a five-year experience. *Am J Gastroenterol* 1999;94(6): 1587–92.

85. D'Haens G, Lemmens L, Geboes K, et al. Intravenous cyclosporine versus intravenous corticosteroids as single therapy for severe attacks of ulcerative colitis. *Gastroenterology* 2001;120(6):1323–29.

86. Van Assche G, D'haens G, Noman M, et al. Randomized, double-blind comparison of 4 mg/kg versus 2 mg/kg intravenous cyclosporine in severe ulcerative colitis. *Gastroenterology* 2003;125(4):1025–31.

87. Arts J, D'Haens G, Zeegers M, et al. Long-term outcome of treatment with intravenous cyclosporin in patients with severe ulcerative colitis. *Inflamm Bowel Dis* 2004;10(2):73–78.

88. Moskovitz DN, Van Assche G, Maenhout B, et al. Incidence of colectomy during long-term follow-up after cyclosporine-induced remission of severe ulcerative colitis. *Clin Gastroenterol Hepatol* 2006;4(6): 760–65.

89. Bressler B, Sands BE. Medical therapy for fistulizing Crohn's disease (Review). *Aliment Pharmacol Ther* 2006;24(9):1283–93.

90. McDonald JW, Feagan BG, Jewell D, et al. Cyclosporine for induction of remission in Crohn's disease. *Cochrane Database Syst Rev* 2005 Apr 18;(2):CD000297.

91. Menachem Y, Gotsman I. Clinical manifestations of pyoderma gangrenosum associated with inflammatory bowel disease. *Isr Med Assoc J* 2004;6(2):88–90.

92. Cat H, Sophani I, Lemann M, et al. Cyclosporin treatment of anal and perianal lesions associated with Crohn's disease. *Turk J Gastroenterol* 2003;14(2):121–27.

93. Hughes AP, Jackson JM, Callen JP. Clinical features and treatment of peristomal pyoderma gangrenosum. *JAMA* 2000;284(12):1546–48.

94. Baumgart DC, Macdonald JK, Feagan B. Tacrolimus (FK506) for induction of remission in refractory ulcerative colitis. *Cochrane Database Syst Rev* 2008;(3):CD007216.

95. Gonzalez-Lama Y, Gisbert JP, Mate J. The role of tacrolimus in inflammatory bowel disease: a systematic review. *Dig Dis Sci* 2006;51(10): 1833–40.

96. Plevy SE, Landers CS, Prehn J, et al. A role for TNF alpha and mucosal T helper-1 cytokines in the pathogenesis of Crohn's disease. *J Immunol* 1997;159(12):6276–82.

97. Van Dullemen HM, Van Deventer SJ, Hommas DW, et al. Treatment of Crohn's disease with anti-tumor necrosis factor chimeric monoclonal antibody (cA2). *Gastroenterology* 1995;109(1):129–35.

98. Targan SR, Hanauer SB, van Deventer SJ, et al. A short term study of chimeric monoclonal antibody cA2 to tumor necrosis factor alpha for Crohn's disease. *N Engl J Med* 1997;337(15):1029–35.

99. D'haens G, Deventer SV, Hogezand RV, et al. Endoscopic and histological healing with Infliximab anti-tumor necrosis factor antibodies in Crohn's disease: a European multicenter trial. *Gastroenterology* 1999; 116(5):1029–34.

100. Present DH, Rutgeerts P, Targan S, et al. Infliximab for the treatment of fistulas in patients with Crohn's disease. *N Engl J Med* 1999; 340(18):1398–405.

101. Rutgeerts P, D'Haens G, Targan S, et al. Efficacy and safety of retreatment with anti-tumor necrosis factor antibody (Infliximab) to maintain remission in Crohn's disease. *Gastroenterology* 1999;117(4): 761–69.

102. Su C, Salzberg BA, Lewis JD, et al. Efficacy of anti-tumor necrosis factor therapy in patients with ulcerative colitis. *Am J Gastroenterol* 2002; 97(10):2577–84.

103. Hanauer SB, Feagan BG, Lichtenstein GR, et al. Maintenance infliximab for Crohn's disease: the ACCENT I randomised trial. *Lancet* 2002; 359(9317):1541–49.

104. Sands BE, Anderson FH, Bernstein CN, et al. Infliximab maintenance therapy for fistulizing Crohn's disease. *N Engl J Med* 2004;350(9): 876–85.

105. Lichtenstein GR, Abreu MT, Cohen R, Tremaine W. American Gastro-enterological Association Institute medical position statement on cortico-steroids, immunomodulators, and infliximab in inflammatory bowel disease. *Gastroenterology* 2006;130(3):935–39.

106. Peyrin-Biroulet L, Deltenre P, De Suray N, et al. Efficacy and safety of tumor necrosis factor antagonists in Crohn's disease: meta-analysis of placebo-controlled trials. *Clin Gastroenterol Hepatol* 2008;6(6):644–53.

107. Behm B, Bickston S. Tumor necrosis factor-alpha antibody for mainte-nance of remission in Crohn's disease. *Cochrane Database Syst Rev* 2008;(1):CD006893.

108. Lemann M, Mary JY, Duclos B, et al. Infliximab plus azathioprine for steroid-dependent Crohn's disease patients: a randomized placebo-con-trolled trial. *Gastroenterology* 2006;130(4):1054–61.

109. Sands BE, Blank MA, Patel K, Van Deventer SJ. Long-term treatment of rectovaginal fistulas in Crohn's disease: response to infliximab in the ACCENT II study. *Clin Gastroenterol Hepatol* 2004;2(10):912–20.

110. Hanauer SB, Sandborn WJ, Rutgeerts P, et al. Human anti-tumor necro-sis factor monoclonal antibody (adalimumab) in Crohn's disease: the CLASSIC-I trial. *Gastroenterology* 2006;130(2):323–33.

111. Sandborn WJ, Hanauer SB, Rutgeerts P, et al. Adalimumab for mainte-nance treatment of Crohn's disease: results of the CLASSIC II trial. *Gut* 2007;56(9):1232–39.

112. Colombel JF, Sandborn WJ, Rutgeerts P, et al. Adalimumab for mainte-nance of clinical response and remission in patients with Crohn's disease: the CHARM trial. *Gastroenterology* 2007;132(1):52–65.

113. Feagan BG, Panaccione R, Sandborn WJ, et al. Effects of adalimumab therapy on incidence of hospitalization and surgery in Crohn's dis-ease: results from the CHARM study. *Gastroenterology* 2008;135(5): 1493–99.

114. Sandborn WJ, Rutgeerts P, Enns R, et al. Adalimumab induction ther-apy for Crohn disease previously treated with infliximab: a randomized trial. *Ann Intern Med* 2007;146(12):829–38.

115. Schreiber S, Rutgeerts P, Fedorak RN, et al. A randomized, placebo-controlled trial of certolizumab pegol (CDP870) for treatment of Crohn's disease. *Gastroenterology* 2005;29(3):807–18.

116. Nesbitt A, Fossati G, Bergin M, et al. Mechanism of action of certolizumab pegol (CDP870): in vitro comparison with other anti-tumor necrosis factor alpha agents. *Inflamm Bowel Dis* 2007;13(11):1323–32.

117. Sandborn WJ, Feagan BG, Stoinov S, et al. Certolizumab pegol for the treatment of Crohn's disease. *N Engl J Med* 2007;357(3):228–38.

118. Schreiber S, Khaliq-Kareemi M, Lawrence IC, et al. Maintenance therapy with certolizumab pegol for Crohn's disease. *N Engl J Med* 2007; 357(3):239–50.

119. Vermeire S, Abreu M, D'Haens G, et al. Efficacy and safety of certolizumab pegol in patients with active Crohn's disease who previously lost response or were intolerant to infliximab: open label induction: preliminary results of the Welcome study (Abstract). *Gastroenterology* 2008; 134(4):A67–68.

120. Rutgeerts P, Feagan BG, Lichtenstein GR, et al. Comparison of scheduled and episodic treatment strategies of infliximab in Crohn's disease. *Gastroenterology* 2004;126(2):402–13.

121. Van Assche G, Magdelaine-Beuzelin C, D'Haens G, et al. Withdrawal of immunosuppression in Crohn's disease treated with scheduled infliximab maintenance: a randomized trial. *Gastroenterology* 2008; 134(7):1861–68.

122. Baert F, Noman M, Vermeire S, et al. Influence of immunogenicity on the long-term efficacy of infliximab in Crohn's disease. *N Engl J Med* 2003;348(7):601–608.

123. Colombel JF, Loftus EV Jr, Tremaine WJ, et al. The safety profile of infliximab in patients with Crohn's disease: the Mayo clinic experience in 500 patients. *Gastroenterology* 2004;126(1):19–31.

124. Biancone L, Calabrese E, Petruzziello C, Pallone F. Treatment with biologic therapies and the risk of cancer in patients with IBD (Review). *Nat Clin Pract Gastroenterol Hepatol* 2007;4(2):78–91.

125. Kwon JH, Farrell RJ. The risk of lymphoma in the treatment of inflammatory bowel disease with immunosuppressive agents (Review). *Crit Rev Oncol Hematol* 2005;56(1):169–78.

126. U.S. lymphoma rates: http://seer.cancer.gov/csr/1975_2006/browse_csr.php?section=19&page=sect_19_table.04.html Accessed 7/25/09.

127. Targan SR, Feagan BG, Fedorak RN, et al., International Efficacy of Natalizumab in Crohn's Disease Response and Remission (ENCORE) Trial Group. Natalizumab for the treatment of active Crohn's disease: results of the ENCORE Trial. *Gastroenterology* 2007;132(5): 1672–83.

128. Sandborn WJ, Colombel JF, Enns R, et al., International Efficacy of Natalizumab as Active Crohn's Therapy (ENACT-1) Trial Group, Evaluation of Natalizumab as Continuous Therapy (ENACT-2) Trial Group. Natalizumab induction and maintenance therapy for Crohn's disease. *N Engl J Med* 2005;353(18):1912–25.

129. Ghosh S, Goldin E, Gordon FH, et al., Natalizumab Pan-European Study Group. Natalizumab for active Crohn's disease. *N Engl J Med* 2003;348(1):24–32.

130. Van Assche G, Van Ranst M, Sciot R, et al. Progressive multifocal leukoencephalopathy after natalizumab therapy for Crohn's disease. *N Engl J Med* 2005;353(4):362–68.

131. Yousry TA, Major EO, Ryschkewitsch C, et al. Evaluation of patients treated with natalizumab for progressive multifocal leukoencephalopathy. *N Engl J Med* 2006;354(9):924–33.

132. Feagan BG, Yan S, Bala M, et al. The effects of infliximab maintenance therapy on health-related quality of life. *Am J Gastroenterol* 2003; 98(10):2232–38.

133. Lichtenstein GR, Yan S, Bala M, et al. Infliximab maintenance treatment reduces hospitalizations, surgeries, and procedures in fistulizing Crohn's disease. *Gastroenterology* 2005;128(4):862–69.

134. Loftus EV, Feagan BG, Colombel JF, et al. Effects of adalimumab maintenance therapy on health-related quality of life of patients with Crohn's

disease: patient-reported outcomes of the CHARM trial. *Am J Gastroenterol* 2008;103(12):3132–41.

135. Rutgeerts P, Schreiber S, Feagan B, et al. Certolizumab pegol, a monthly subcutaneously administered Fc-free anti-TNFalpha, improves health-related quality of life in patients with moderate to severe Crohn's disease. *Int J Colorectal Dis* 2008;23(3):289–96.

136. Siegel CA, Levy LC, Mackenzie TA, Sands BE. Patient perceptions of the risks and benefits of infliximab for the treatment of inflammatory bowel disease. *Inflamm Bowel Dis* 2008;14(1):1–6.

137. Johnson FR, Ozdemir S, Mansfield C, et al. Crohn's disease patients' risk-benefit preferences: serious adverse event risks versus treatment efficacy. *Gastroenterology* 2007;133(3):769–79.

138. Kane S, Stone LJ, Ehrenpreis E. Thalidomide as "salvage" therapy for patients with delayed hypersensitivity response to infliximab: a case series. *J Clin Gastroenterol* 2002;35(2):149–50.

139. Sabate JM, Villarejo J, Lemann M, et al. An open-label study of thalidomide for maintenance therapy in responders to infliximab in chronically active and fistulizing refractory Crohn's disease. *Aliment Pharmacol Ther* 2002;16(6):1117–24.

140. Vasiliauskas EA, Kam LY, Abreu-Martin MT, et al. An open-label pilot study of low-dose thalidomide in chronically active, steroid-dependent Crohn's disease. *Gastroenterology* 1999;117(6):1278–87.

141. Ehrenpreis ED, Kane SV, Cohen LB, et al. Thalidomide therapy for patients with refractory Crohn's disease: an open-label trial. *Gastroenterology* 1999;117(6):1271–77.

142. Mansfield JC, Parkes M, Hawthorne AB, et al. A randomized, double-blind, placebo-controlled trial of lenalidomide in the treatment of moderately severe active Crohn's disease. *Aliment Pharmacol Ther* 2007; 26(3):421–30.

143. Pardi DS, Loftus EV Jr, Camilleri M. Treatment of inflammatory bowel disease in the elderly: an update. *Drugs Aging* 2002;19(5): 355–63.

144. Takeuchi K, Smale S, Premchand P, et al. Prevalence and mechanism of nonsteroidal anti-inflammatory drug-induced clinical relapse in patients with inflammatory bowel disease. *Clin Gastroenterol Hepatol* 2006; 4(2):196–202.

145. Meyer AM, Ramzan NN, Heigh RI, Leighton JA. Relapse of inflammatory bowel disease associated with use of nonsteroidal anti-inflammatory drugs. *Dig Dis Sci* 2006;51(1):168–72.

146. Felder JB, Korelitz BI, Rajapakse R, et al. Effects of nonsteroidal anti-inflammatory drugs on inflammatory bowel disease: a case-control study. *Am J Gastroenterol* 2000;95(8):1949–54.

147. Lewis JD, Lichtenstein GR, Deren JJ, et al. Rosiglitazone for active ulcerative colitis: a randomized placebo-controlled trial. *Gastroenterology* 2008; 134(3):688–95.

148. Stremmel W, Ehehalt R, Autschbach F, Karner M. Phosphatidylcholine for steroid-refractory chronic ulcerative colitis: a randomized trial. *Ann Intern Med* 2007;147(9):603–10.

149. Feagan BG, Greenberg GR, Wild G, et al. Treatment of ulcerative colitis with a humanized antibody to the alpha4beta7 integrin. *N Engl J Med* 2005;352(24):2499–507.

150. Tsujikawa T, Andoh A, Ogawa A, et al. Feasibility of five days of consecutive leukocytapheresis for the treatment of ulcerative colitis: a preliminary study. *Ther Apher Dial* 2009;13(1):14–18.

151. Bresci G, Parisi G, Mazzoni A, et al. Granulocytapheresis versus methylprednisolone in patients with acute ulcerative colitis: 12-month follow up. *J Gastroenterol Hepatol* 2008;23(11):1678–82.

152. Sakata Y, Iwakiri R, Amemori S, et al. Comparison of the efficacy of granulocyte and monocyte/macrophage adsorptive apheresis and leukocytapheresis in active ulcerative colitis patients: a prospective randomized study. *Eur J Gastroenterol Hepatol* 2008;20(7): 629–33.

153. Sands BE, Sandborn WJ, Feagan B, et al., Adacolumn Study Group. A randomized, double-blind, sham-controlled study of granulocyte/

monocyte apheresis for active ulcerative colitis. *Gastroenterology* 2008; 135(2):400–409.

154. Akobeng AK, Thomas AG. Enteral nutrition for maintenance of remission in Crohn's disease. *Cochrane Database Syst Rev* 2007;(3): CD005984.

155. Ostro MJ, Greenberg GR, Jeejebhoy KN. Total parenteral nutrition and complete bowel rest in the management of Crohn's disease. *J Parenter Enteral Nutr* 1985;9(3):280–287.

156. Fukuda Y, Takazoe M, Sugita A, et al. Oral spherical adsorptive carbon for the treatment of intractable anal fistulas in Crohn's disease: a multi-center, randomized, double-blind, placebo-controlled trial. *Am J Gastroenterol* 2008;103(7):1721–29.

157. Calenda KA, Schornagel IL, Sadeghi-Nejad A, Grand RJ. Effect of recombinant growth hormone treatment on children with Crohn's disease and short stature: a pilot study. *Inflamm Bowel Dis* 2005;11(5): 435–41.

158. Slonim AE, Bulone L, Damore MB, et al. A preliminary study of growth hormone therapy for Crohn's disease. *N Engl J Med* 2000;342(22): 1633–37.

159. Garcia-Olmo D, Herreros D, Pascual M, et al. Treatment of enterocutaneous fistula in Crohn's disease with adipose-derived stem cells: a comparison of protocols with and without cell expansion. *Int J Colorectal Dis* 2009;24(1):27–30.

160. Cassinotti A, Annaloro C, Ardizzone S, et al. Autologous haematopoietic stem cell transplantation without CD34+ cell selection in refractory Crohn's disease. *Gut* 2008;57(2):211–17.

161. García-Olmo D, García-Arranz M, Herreros D, et al. A phase I clinical trial of the treatment of Crohn's fistula by adipose mesenchymal stem cell transplantation. *Dis Colon Rectum* 2005;48(7):1416–23.

162. Korzenik JR, Dieckgraefe BK, Valentine JF, et al., Sargramostim in Crohn's Disease Study Group. Sargramostim for active Crohn's disease. *N Engl J Med* 2005;352(21):2193–201.

163. Smith JP, Stock H, Bingaman S, et al. Low-dose naltrexone therapy improves active Crohn's disease. *Am J Gastroenterol* 2007;102(4): 820–28.

164. Treton X, Bouhnik Y, Mary JY, et al., Groupe D'Etude Thérapeutique Des Affections Inflammatoires Du Tube Digestif (GETAID). Azathioprine withdrawal in patients with Crohn's disease maintained on prolonged remission: a high risk of relapse. *Clin Gastroenterol Hepatol* 2009;7(1):80–85.

165. Lichtenstein GR, Yan S, Bala M, Hanauer S. Remission in patients with Crohn's disease is associated with improvement in employment and quality of life and a decrease in hospitalizations and surgeries. *Am J Gastroenterol* 2004;99(1):91–96.

166. Kane S, Huo D, Aikens J, Hanauer S. Medication nonadherence and the outcomes of patients with quiescent ulcerative colitis. *Am J Med* 2003;114(1):39–43.

167. Higgins PD, Rubin DT, Kaulback K, et al. Systematic review: impact of non-adherence to 5-aminosalicylic acid products on the frequency and cost of ulcerative colitis flares. *Aliment Pharmacol Ther* 2009;29(3): 247–57.

168. Kane S, Shaya F. Medication non-adherence is associated with increased medical health care costs. *Dig Dis Sci* 2008;53(4):1020–24.

169. Sewitch MJ, Abrahamowicz M, Barkun A, et al. Patient nonadherence to medication in inflammatory bowel disease. *Am J Gastroenterol* 2003; 98(7):1535–44.

170. Wong AP, Clark AL, Garnett EA, et al. Use of complementary medicine in pediatric patients with inflammatory bowel disease: results from a multicenter survey. *J Pediatr Gastroenterol Nutr* 2009;48(1):55–60.

171. Rahimi R, Mozaffari S, Abdollahi M. On the use of herbal medicines in management of inflammatory bowel diseases: a systematic review of animal and human studies. *Dig Dis Sci* 2009;54(3):471–80.

172. Langhorst J, Anthonisen IB, Steder-Neukamm U, et al. Patterns of complementary and alternative medicine (CAM) use in patients with inflam-

matory bowel disease: perceived stress is a potential indicator for CAM use. *Complement Ther Med* 2007;15(1):30–37.

173. Joos S, Rosemann T, Szecsenyi J, et al. Use of complementary and alternative medicine in Germany: a survey of patients with inflammatory bowel disease. *BMC Complement Altern Med* 2006;6:19.

174. Li FX, Verhoef MJ, Best A, et al. Why patients with inflammatory bowel disease use or do not use complementary and alternative medicine: a Canadian national survey. *Can J Gastroenterol* 2005;19(9):567–73.

175. Bensoussan M, Jovenin N, Garcia B, et al. Complementary and alternative medicine use by patients with inflammatory bowel disease: results from a postal survey. *Gastroenterol Clin Biol* 2006;30(1):14–23.

176. Hilsden RJ, Verhoef MJ, Best A, Pocobelli G. Complementary and alternative medicine use by Canadian patients with inflammatory bowel disease: results from a national survey. *Am J Gastroenterol* 2003;98(7): 1563–68.

177. Quattropani C, Ausfeld B, Straumann A, et al. Comple-mentary alternative medicine in patients with inflammatory bowel disease: use and attitudes. *Scand J Gastroenterol* 2003;38(3):277–82.

178. Leung VW, Shalansky SJ, Lo MK, Jadusingh EA. Prevalence of use and the risk of adverse effects associated with complementary and alternative medicine in a cohort of patients receiving warfarin. *Ann Pharmacother* 2009;43(5):875–81.

179. Aslan A, Triadafilopoulos G. Fish oil fatty acid supplementation in active ulcerative colitis: a double-blind, placebo-controlled, crossover study. *Am J Gastroenterol* 1992;87(4):432–37.

180. Stenson WF, Cort D, Rodgers J, et al. Dietary supplementation with fish oil in ulcerative colitis. *Ann Intern Med* 1992;116(8):609–14.

181. Lorenz-Meyer H, Bauer P, Nicolay C, et al., Study Group Members (German Crohn's Disease Study Group). Omega-3 fatty acids and low carbohydrate diet for maintenance of remission in Crohn's disease: a randomized controlled multicenter trial. *Scand J Gastroenterol* 1996;31(8): 778–85.

182. Belluzzi A, Brignola C, Campieri M, et al. Effect of an enteric-coated fish-oil preparation on relapses in Crohn's disease. *N Engl J Med* 1996; 334(24):1557–60.

183. Seidner DL, Lashner BA, Brzezinski A, et al. An oral supplement enriched with fish oil, soluble fiber, and antioxidants for corticosteroid sparing in ulcerative colitis: a randomized, controlled trial. *Clin Gastroenterol Hepatol* 2005;3(4):358–69.

184. Romano C, Cucchiara S, Barabino A, et al. Usefulness of omega-3 fatty acid supplementation in addition to mesalazine in maintaining remission in pediatric Crohn's disease: a double-blind, randomized, placebo-controlled study. *World J Gastroenterol* 2005;11(45):7118–21.

185. Turner D, Steinhart AH, Griffiths AM. Omega 3 fatty acids (fish oil) for maintenance of remission in ulcerative colitis. *Cochrane Database Syst Rev* 2007;(3):CD006443.

186. Feagan BG, Sandborn WJ, Mittmann U, et al. Omega-3 free fatty acids for the maintenance of remission in Crohn disease: the EPIC Randomized Controlled Trials. *JAMA* 2008;299(14):1690–97.

187. Holt PR, Katz S, Kirshoff R. Curcumin therapy in inflammatory bowel disease: a pilot study. *Dig Dis Sci* 2005;50(11):2191–93.

188. Hanai H, Iida T, Takeuchi K, et al. Curcumin maintenance therapy for ulcerative colitis: randomized, multicenter, double-blind, placebo-controlled trial. *Clin Gastroenterol Hepatol* 2006;4(12): 1502–506.

189. Borkow G, Leng Q, Weisman Z, et al. Chronic immune activation associated with intestinal helminth infections results in impaired signal transduction and anergy. *J Clin Invest* 2000;106(8):1053–60.

190. Summers RW, Elliott DE, Urban JF Jr, et al. Trichuris suis therapy for active ulcerative colitis: a randomized controlled trial. *Gastroenterology* 2005;128(4):825–32.

191. Chapman TM, Plosker GL, Figgitt DP. VSL#3 probiotic mixture: a review of its use in chronic inflammatory bowel diseases (Review). *Drugs* 2006;66(10):1371–87.

192. Fujimori S, Gudis K, Mitsui K, et al. A randomized controlled trial on the efficacy of symbiotic versus probiotic or prebiotic treatment to improve the quality of life in patients with ulcerative colitis. *Nutrition* 2009;25(5):520–25.

193. Miele E, Pascarella F, Giannetti E, et al. Effect of a probiotic preparation (VSL#3) on induction and maintenance of remission in children with ulcerative colitis. *Am J Gastroenterol* 2009;104(2): 437–43.

194. Butterworth AD, Thomas AG, Akobeng AK. Probiotics for induction of remission in Crohn's disease (Review). *Cochrane Database Syst Rev* 2008 Jul 16;(3):CD006634.

195. Garcia Vilela E, De Lourdes De Abreu Ferrari M, Oswaldo Da Gama Torres H, et al. Influence of Saccharomyces boulardii on the intestinal permeability of patients with Crohn's disease in remission. *Scand J Gastroenterol* 2008;43(7):842–48.

196. Tursi A. Balsalazide plus high-potency probiotic preparation (VSL#3) in the treatment of acute mild-to-moderate ulcerative colitis and uncomplicated diverticulitis of the colon (Review). *J Clin Gastroenterol* 2008;42 (Suppl. 3, Pt. 1):S119–22.

197. Henker J, Müller S, Laass MW, et al. Probiotic *Escherichia coli* Nissle 1917 (EcN) for successful remission maintenance of ulcerative colitis in children and adolescents: an open-label pilot study. *Z Gastroenterol* 2008;46(9):874–75.

198. Schultz M. Clinical use of *E. coli* Nissle 1917 in inflammatory bowel disease (Review). *Inflamm Bowel Dis* 2008;14(7):1012–18.

199. Kruis W, Fric P, Pokrotnieks J, et al. Maintaining remission of ulcerative colitis with the probiotic *Escherichia coli* Nissle 1917 is as effective as with standard mesalazine. *Gut* 2004;53(11):1617–23.

200. Rembacken BJ, Snelling AM, Hawkey PM, Chalmers DM, Axon AT. Non-pathogenic *Escherichia coli* versus mesalazine for the treatment of ulcerative colitis: a randomised trial. *Lancet* 1999;354(9179): 635–39.

201. Kruis W, Schütz E, Fric P, et al. Double-blind comparison of an oral *Escherichia coli* preparation and mesalazine in maintaining remission of ulcerative colitis. *Aliment Pharmacol Ther* 1997;11(5):853–58.

202. Loftus EV Jr. Management of extraintestinal manifestations and other complications of inflammatory bowel disease (Review). *Curr Gastroenterol Rep* 2004;6(6):506–13.

203. Patel H, Barr A, Jeejeebhoy KN. Renal effects of long-term treatment with 5-aminosalicylic acid. *Can J Gastroenterol* 2009;23(3):170–76.

204. Ali T, Lam D, Bronze MS, Humphrey MB. Osteoporosis in inflammatory bowel disease (Review). *Am J Med* 2009;122(7):599–604.

205. Bernstein CN, Blanchard JF, Leslie W, et al. The incidence of fracture among patients with inflammatory bowel disease: a population-based cohort study. *Ann Intern Med* 2000;133(10):795–99.

206. Palomba S, Manguso F, Orio F Jr, et al. Effectiveness of risedronate in osteoporotic postmenopausal women with inflammatory bowel disease: a prospective, parallel, open-label, two-year extension study. *Menopause* 2008;15(4, Pt. 1):730–36.

207. Kitazaki S, Mitsuyama K, Masuda J, et al. Clinical trial: comparison of alendronate and alfacalcidol in glucocorticoid-associated osteoporosis in patients with ulcerative colitis. *Aliment Pharmacol Ther* 2009;29(4):424–30.

208. Hart AL, Plamondon S, Kamm MA. Topical tacrolimus in the treatment of perianal Crohn's disease: exploratory randomized controlled trial. *Inflamm Bowel Dis* 2007;13(3):245–53.

209. U.S. colon cancer rates: http://seer.cancer.gov/csr/1975_2006/browse_csr.php?section=6&page=sect_06_table.05.html. Accessed 7/25/09.

210. Jess T, Loftus EV Jr, Velayos FS, et al. Incidence and prognosis of colorectal dysplasia in inflammatory bowel disease: a population-based study from Olmsted County, Minnesota. *Inflamm Bowel Dis* 2006;12(8):669–76.

211. Triantafillidis JK, Nasioulas G, Kosmidis PA. Colorectal cancer and inflammatory bowel disease: epidemiology, risk factors, mechanisms of

carcinogenesis and prevention strategies. *Anticancer Res* 2009;29(7): 2727–37.

212. Friedman S, Rubin PH, Bodian C, et al. Screening and surveillance colonoscopy in chronic Crohn's colitis: results of a surveillance program spanning 25 years. *Clin Gastroenterol Hepatol* 2008;6(9): 993–98.

213. Haskell H, Andrews CW Jr, Reddy SI, et al. Pathologic features and clinical significance of "backwash" ileitis in ulcerative colitis. *Am J Surg Pathol* 2005;29(11):1472–81.

214. Friedman S, Odze RD, Farraye FA. Management of neoplastic polyps in inflammatory bowel disease (Review). *Inflamm Bowel Dis* 2003; 9(4):260–66.

215. Rubin PH, Friedman S, Harpaz N, et al. Colonoscopic polypectomy in chronic colitis: conservative management after endoscopic resection of dysplastic polyps. *Gastroenterology* 1999;117(6):1295–300.

216. Lashner, BA, Provencher, KS, Seidner, DL, et al. The effect of folic acid supplementation on the risk for cancer or dysplasia in ulcerative colitis. *Gastroenterology* 1997;112(1):29–32.

217. Wolf JM, Rybicki LA, Lashner BA. The impact of ursodeoxycholic acid on cancer, dysplasia and mortality in ulcerative colitis patients with primary sclerosing cholangitis. *Aliment Pharmacol Ther* 2005;22(9): 783–88.

218. Pardi DS, Loftus EV Jr, Kremers WK, et al. Urso-deoxycholic acid as a chemopreventive agent in patients with ulcerative colitis and primary sclerosing cholangitis. *Gastroenterology* 2003;124(4):889–93.

219. Beaugerie L, Carrat F, Bouvier AM, et al., for the CESAME study group. Excess risk of lymphoproliferative disorders (LPD) in inflammatory bowel diseases (IBD): interim results of the Cesame cohort. *Gastroenterology* 2008;134(4):A116–17.

220. Mackey AC, Green L, Liang LC, et al. Hepatosplenic T cell lymphoma associated with infliximab use in young patients treated for inflammatory bowel disease. *J Pediatr Gastroenterol Nutr* 2007;44(2):265–67.

221. Burger DC, Florin TH. Hepatosplenic T-cell lymphoma following infliximab therapy for Crohn's disease. *Med J Aust* 2009;190(6): 341–42.

222. Mackey AC, Green L, Leptak C, Avigan M. Hepatosplenic T cell lymphoma associated with infliximab use in young patients treated for inflammatory bowel disease: update. *J Pediatr Gastroenterol Nutr* 2009; 48(3):386–88.

223. Jess T, Loftus EV Jr, Velayos FS, et al. Risk of intestinal cancer in inflammatory bowel disease: a population-based study from Olmsted County, Minnesota. *Gastroenterology* 2006;130(4):1039–46.

224. Piton G, Cosnes J, Monnet E, et al. Risk factors associated with small bowel adenocar-cinoma in Crohn's disease: a case-control study. *Am J Gastroenterol* 2008;103(7):1730–36.

225. Sampietro GM, Corsi F, Maconi G, et al. Prospective study of long-term results and prognostic factors after conservative surgery for small bowel Crohn's disease. *Clin Gastroenterol Hepatol* 2009;7(2):183–91.

226. Shen B, Remzi FH, Lavery IC, et al. A proposed classification of ileal pouch disorders and associated complications after restorative proctocolectomy. *Clin Gastroenterol Hepatol* 2008;6(2):145–58.

227. Shen B, Lashner BA, Bennett AE, et al. Treatment of rectal cuff inflammation (cuffitis) in patients with ulcerative colitis following restorative proctocolectomy and ileal pouch-anal anastomosis. *Am J Gastroenterol* 2004;99(8):1527–31.

228. Shen B, Fazio VW, Remzi FH, et al. Risk factors for diseases of ileal pouch-anal anastomosis after restorative proctocolectomy for ulcerative colitis. *Clin Gastroenterol Hepatol* 2006;4(1):81–89.

229. Mimura T, Rizzello F, Helwig U, et al. Once daily high dose probiotic therapy (VSL#3) for maintaining remission in recurrent or refractory pouchitis. *Gut* 2004;53(1):108–14.

230. Gionchetti P, Rizzello F, Helwig U, et al., Campieri M. Prophylaxis of pouchitis onset with probiotic therapy: a double-blind, placebo-controlled trial. *Gastroenterology* 2003;124(5):1202–209.

231. Wu H, Shen B. Crohn's disease of the pouch: diagnosis and management (Review). *Expert Rev Gastroenterol Hepatol* 2009;3(2):155–65.

232. Berndtsson I, Lindholm E, Oresland T, Börjesson L. Long-term outcome after ileal pouch-anal anastomosis: function and health-related quality of life. *Dis Colon Rectum* 2007;50(10):1545–52.

233. Hahnloser D, Pemberton JH, Wolff BG, et al. Results at up to 20 years after ileal pouch-anal anastomosis for chronic ulcerative colitis. *Br J Surg* 2007;94(3):333–40.

234. Jowett SL, Seal CJ, Pearce MS, et al. Influence of dietary factors on the clinical course of ulcerative colitis: a prospective cohort study. *Gut* 2004; 53(10):1479–84.

235. Fernandez-Banares F, Hinojosa J, Sanchez-Lombrana L, et al. Randomized clinical trial of Plantago ovata seeds (dietary fiber) as compared with mesalamine in maintaining remission in ulcerative colitis. *Am J Gastroenterol* 1999;94(2):427–33.

236. Lecleire S, Hassan A, Marion-Letellier R, et al. Combined glutamine and arginine decrease proinflammatory cytokine production by biopsies from Crohn's patients in association with changes in nuclear factor-kappaB and p38 mitogen-activated protein kinase pathways. *J Nutr* 2008; 138(12):2481–86.

237. Kanauchi O, Mitsuyama K, Homma T, et al. Treatment of ulcerative colitis patients by long-term administration of germinated barley foodstuff: multi-center open trial. *Int J Mol Med* 2003;12(5):701–704.

238. Akobeng AK, Miller V, Stanton J, et al. Double-blind randomized controlled trial of glutamine-enriched polymeric diet in the treatment of active Crohn's disease. *J Pediatr Gastroenterol Nutr* 2000;30(1): 78–84.

239. Smith PA. Nutritional therapy for active Crohn's disease (Review). *World J Gastroenterol* 2008;14(27):4420–23.

240. Issa M, Binion DG. Bowel rest and nutrition therapy in the management of active Crohn's disease (Review). *Nutr Clin Pract* 2008;23(3): 299–308.

241. Yamamoto T, Nakahigashi M, Saniabadi AR, et al. Impacts of long-term enteral nutrition on clinical and endoscopic disease activities and mucosal cytokines during remission in patients with Crohn's disease: a prospective study. *Inflamm Bowel Dis* 2007;13(12):1493–501.

242. Evans JP, Steinhart AH, Cohen Z, McLeod RS. Home total parenteral nutrition: an alternative to early surgery for complicated inflammatory bowel disease. *J Gastrointest Surg* 2003;7(4):562–66.

243. Campos FG, Waitzberg DL, Teixeira MG, et al. Pharmacological nutrition in inflammatory bowel diseases. *Nutr Hosp* 2003;18(2):57–64.

244. Seo M, Okada M, Yao T, et al. The role of total parenteral nutrition in the management of patients with acute attacks of inflammatory bowel disease. *J Clin Gastroenterol* 1999;29(3):270–75.

245. Bitton, A, Sewitch, MJ, Peppercorn, MA, et al. Psychosocial determinants of relapse in ulcerative colitis: a longitudinal study. *Am J Gastroenterol* 2003;98(10):2203–208.

246. Li J, Nørgard B, Precht DH, Olsen J. Psychological stress and inflammatory bowel disease: a follow-up study in parents who lost a child in Denmark. *Am J Gastroenterol* 2004;99(6):1129–33.

247. Maunder RG, Levenstein S. The role of stress in the development and clinical course of inflammatory bowel disease: epidemiological evidence (Review). *Curr Mol Med* 2008;8(4):247–52.

248. Bernstein CN, Walker JR, Graff LA. On studying the connection between stress and IBD. *Am J Gastroenterol* 2006;101(4):782–85.

249. Lerebours E, Gower-Rousseau C, Merle V, et al. Stressful life events as a risk factor for inflammatory bowel disease onset: a population-based case-control study. *Am J Gastroenterol* 2007;102(1):122–31.

250. Reese GE, Nanidis T, Borysiewicz C, et al. The effect of smoking after surgery for Crohn's disease: a meta-analysis of observational studies. *Int J Colorectal Dis* 2008;23(12):1213–21.

251. Ernst A, Jacobsen B, Østergaard M, et al. Mutations in CARD15 and smoking confer susceptibility to Crohn's disease in the Danish population. *Scand J Gastroenterol* 2007;42(12):1445–51.

252. Tuvlin JA, Raza SS, Bracamonte S, et al. Smoking and inflammatory bowel disease: trends in familial and sporadic cohorts. *Inflamm Bowel Dis* 2007;13(5):573–79.

253. Mahid SS, Minor KS, Stromberg AJ, Galandiuk S. Active and passive smoking in childhood is related to the development of inflammatory bowel disease. *Inflamm Bowel Dis* 2007;13(4):431–38.

254. Cosnes J, Nion-Larmurier I, Afchain P, et al. Gender differences in the response of colitis to smoking. *Clin Gastroenterol Hepatol* 2004; 2(1):41–48.

255. Van der Heide F, Dijkstra A, Weersma RK, et al. Effects of active and passive smoking on disease course of Crohn's disease and ulcerative colitis. *Inflamm Bowel Dis* 2009;15(8):1199–207.

256. Pullan RD, Rhodes J, Ganesh S, et al. Transdermal nicotine for active ulcerative colitis. *N Engl J Med* 1994;330(12):811–15.

257. Sandborn WJ, Tremaine W, Offord KP, et al. Transdermal nicotine for mildly to moderately active ulcerative colitis: a randomized, double-blind, placebo-controlled trial. *Ann Intern Med* 1997;126(5): 364–71.

258. Thomas GA, Rhodes J, Ragunath K, et al. Transdermal nicotine compared with oral prednisolone therapy for active ulcerative colitis. *Eur J Gastroenterol Hepatol* 1996;8(8):769–76.

259. Thomas GA, Rhodes J, Mani V, et al. Transdermal nicotine as maintenance therapy for ulcerative colitis. *N Engl J Med* 1995;332(15): 988–92.

260. Orel R, Kamhi T, Vidmar G, Mamula P. Epidemiology of pediatric chronic inflammatory bowel disease in central and western Slovenia, 1994–2005. *J Pediatr Gastroenterol Nutr* 2009;48(5):579–86.

261. Kugathasan S, Judd RH, Hoffmann RG, et al., Wisconsin Pediatric Inflammatory Bowel Disease Alliance. Epidemiologic and clinical characteristics of children with newly diagnosed inflammatory bowel disease in Wisconsin: a statewide population-based study. *J Pediatr* 2003; 143(4):525–31.

262. Perminow G, Brackmann S, Lyckander LG, et al., IBSEN-II Group. A characterization in childhood inflammatory bowel disease, a new population-based inception cohort from southeastern Norway, 2005–07, showing increased incidence in Crohn's disease. *Scand J Gastroenterol* 2009;44(4):446–56.

263. Vernier-Massouille G, Balde M, Salleron J, et al. Natural history of pediatric Crohn's disease: a population-based cohort study. *Gastroenterology* 2008;135(4):1106–13.

264. Castro M, Papadatou B, Baldassare M, et al. Inflammatory bowel disease in children and adolescents in Italy: data from the pediatric national IBD register (1996–2003). *Inflamm Bowel Dis* 2008;14(9):1246–52.

265. Otley AR, Griffiths AM, Hale S, et al., Pediatric IBD Collaborative Research Group. Health-related quality of life in the first year after a diagnosis of pediatric inflammatory bowel disease. *Inflamm Bowel Dis* 2006;12(8):684–91.

266. Grossman AB, Baldassano RN. Specific considerations in the treatment of pediatric inflammatory bowel disease (Review). *Expert Rev Gastroenterol Hepatol* 2008;2(1):105–24.

267. Maunder RG, Greenberg GR, Lancee WJ, et al. The impact of ulcerative colitis is greater in unmarried and young patients. *Can J Gastroenterol* 2007;21(11):715–20.

268. Dubinsky MC, Lin YC, Dutridge D, et al., Western Regional Pediatric IBD Research Alliance. Serum immune responses predict rapid disease progression among children with Crohn's disease: immune responses predict disease progression. *Am J Gastroenterol* 2006;101(2):360–67.

269. Hyams J, Markowitz J, Lerer T, et al., Pediatric Inflammatory Bowel Disease Collaborative Research Group. The natural history of corticosteroid therapy for ulcerative colitis in children. *Clin Gastroenterol Hepatol* 2006;4(9):1118–23.

270. Punati J, Markowitz J, Lerer T, et al., Pediatric IBD Collaborative Research Group. Effect of early immunomodulator use in moderate to severe pediatric Crohn disease. *Inflamm Bowel Dis* 2008;14(7):949–54.

271. Markowitz J, Grancher K, Mandel F, Daum F, Subcommittee on Immunosuppressive Use of the Pediatric IBD Collaborative Research Forum. Immunosuppressive therapy in pediatric inflammatory bowel disease: results of a survey of the North American Society for Pediatric Gastroenterology and Nutrition. *Am J Gastroenterol* 1993;88(1):44–48.

272. Hyams J, Crandall W, Kugathasan S, et al., REACH Study Group. Induction and maintenance infliximab therapy for the treatment of moderate-to-severe Crohn's disease in children. *Gastroenterology* 2007; 132(3):863–73.

273. Kugathasan S, Werlan SL, Aktay N, et al. Prolonged duration of response to infliximab in early pediatric Crohn's disease (CD): one year follow up (Abstract). *Gastroenterology* 2000;118:A566.

274. Vasiliauskas EA, Schaffer S, Dezenberg CV, et al. Collaborative experience of open-label infliximab in refractory pediatric Crohn's disease (Abstract). *Gastroenterology* 2000;118:A178.

275. Stephens MC, Shepanski MA, Mamula P, et al. Safety and steroid-sparing experience using infliximab for Crohn's disease at a pediatric inflammatory bowel disease center. *Am J Gastroenterol* 2003;98(1): 104–11.

276. Baldassano R, Braegger CP, Escher JC, DeWoody K. Infliximab (Remicade) therapy in the treatment of pediatric Crohn's disease. *Am J Gastroenterol* 2003;98(4):833–38.

277. De Ridder L, Escher JC, Bouquet J, et al. Infliximab therapy in 30 patients with refractory pediatric Crohn disease with and without fistulas in The Netherlands. *J Pediatr Gastroenterol Nutr* 2004;39(1):46–52.

278. Markowitz J, Hyams J, Mack D, et al. Corticosteroid therapy in the age of infliximab: acute and 1-year outcomes in newly diagnosed children with Crohn's disease. *Clin Gastroenterol Hepatol* 2006;4(9): 1124–29.

279. Hyams J, Crandall W, Kugathasan S, et al. Induction and maintenance infliximab therapy for the treatment of moderate-to-severe Crohn's disease in children. *Gastroenterology* 2007;132(2):863–73.

280. Thayu M, Leonard MB, Hyams JS, et al., REACH Study Group. Improvement in biomarkers of bone formation during infliximab therapy in pediatric Crohn's disease: results of the REACH study. *Clin Gastroenterol Hepatol* 2008;6(12):1378–84.

281. Wyneski MJ, Green A, Kay M, et al. Safety and efficacy of adalimumab in pediatric patients with Crohn disease. *J Pediatr Gastroenterol Nutr* 2008;47(1):19–25.

282. Hyams JS, Wilson DC, Thomas A, et al., International Natalizumab CD305 Trial Group. Natalizumab therapy for moderate to severe Crohn disease in adolescents. *J Pediatr Gastroenterol Nutr* 2007;44(2):185–91.

283. Thayu M, Markowitz JE, Mamula P, et al. Hepatosplenic T-cell lymphoma in an adolescent patient after immunomodulator and biologic therapy for Crohn disease. *J Pediatr Gastroenterol Nutr* 2005;40(2): 220–22.

284. Mackey AC, Green L, Leptak C, Avigan M. Hepatosplenic T cell lymphoma associated with infliximab use in young patients treated for inflammatory bowel disease: update. *J Pediatr Gastroenterol Nutr* 2009; 48(3):386–88.

285. Drini M, Prichard PJ, Brown GJ, Macrae FA. Hepatosplenic T-cell lymphoma following infliximab therapy for Crohn's disease. *Med J Aust* 2008;189(8):464–65.

286. Shale M, Kanfer E, Panaccione R, Ghosh S. Hepatosplenic T cell lymphoma in inflammatory bowel disease. *Gut* 2008;57(12):1639–41.

287. Rosh JR, Gross T, Mamula P, et al. Hepatosplenic T-cell lymphoma in adolescents and young adults with Crohn's disease: a cautionary tale (Review)? *Inflamm Bowel Dis* 2007;13(8):1024–30.

288. Waljee A, Waljee J, Morris A, Higgins PD. Threefold increased risk of infertility: a meta-analysis of infertility after ileal pouch anal anastomosis in ulcerative colitis. *Gut* 2006;55:1575–80.

289. Peloquin JM, Pardi DS, Sandborn WJ, et al. Diagnostic ionizing radiation exposure in a population-based cohort of patients with inflammatory bowel disease. *Am J Gastroenterol* 2008;103(8):2015–22.

290. Desmond AN, O'Regan K, Curran C, et al. Crohn's disease: factors associated with exposure to high levels of diagnostic radiation. *Gut* 2008; 57(11):1524–29.

291. Gaca AM, Jaffe TA, Delaney S, et al. Radiation doses from small-bowel follow-through and abdomen/pelvis MDCT in pediatric Crohn disease. *Pediatr Radiol* 2008;38(3):285–91.

292. Jaffe TA, Gaca AM, Delaney S, et al. Radiation doses from small-bowel follow-through and abdominopelvic MDCT in Crohn's disease. *Am J Roentgenol* 2007;189(5):1015–22.

293. Greenley RN, Stephens M, Doughty A, et al. Barriers to adherence among adolescents with inflammatory bowel disease. *Inflamm Bowel Dis* 2010;16(1):36–41.

294. Maunder R, Toner B, de Rooy E, Moskovitz D. Influence of sex and disease on illness-related concerns in inflammatory bowel disease. *Can J Gastroenterol* 1999;13(9):728–32.

295. Feagins LA, Kane SV. Sexual and reproductive issues for men with inflammatory bowel disease. *Am J Gastroenterol* 2009;104(3): 768–73.

296. Rajapakse RO, Korelitz BI, Zlatanic J, et al. Outcome of pregnancies when fathers are treated with 6-mercaptopurine for inflammatory bowel disease. *Am J Gastroenterol* 2000;95(3):684–88.

297. Francella A, Dyan A, Bodian C, et al. The safety of 6-mercaptopurine for childbearing patients with inflammatory bowel disease: a retrospective cohort study. *Gastroenterology* 2003;124(1):9–17.

298. Nørgård B, Pedersen L, Jacobsen J, et al. The risk of congenital abnormalities in children fathered by men treated with azathioprine or mercaptopurine before conception. *Aliment Pharmacol Ther* 2004;19(6): 679–85.

299. Dejaco C, Mittermaier C, Reinisch W, et al. Azathioprine treatment and male fertility in inflammatory bowel disease. *Gastroenterology* 2001; 121(5):1048–53.

300. Kane SV, Sable K, Hanauer SB. The menstrual cycle and its effect on inflammatory bowel disease and irritable bowel syndrome: a prevalence study. *Am J Gastroenterol* 1998;93(10):1867–72.

301. Lichtarowicz A, Norman C, Calcraft B, et al. A study of the menopause, smoking, and contraception in women with Crohn's disease. *Q J Med* 1989;72(267):623–31.

302. Kane SV, Reddy D. Hormonal replacement therapy after menopause is protective of disease activity in women with inflammatory bowel disease. *Am J Gastroenterol* 2008;103(5):1193–96.

303. Kane S, Khatibi B, Reddy D. Higher incidence of abnormal Pap smears in women with inflammatory bowel disease. *Am J Gastroenterol* 2008; 103(3):631–36.

304. Hutfless S, Fireman B, Kane S, Herrinton LJ. Screening differences and risk of cervical cancer in inflammatory bowel disease. *Aliment Pharmacol Ther* 2008;28(5):598–605.

305. Cornish JA, Tan E, Simillis C, et al. The risk of oral contraceptives in the etiology of inflammatory bowel disease: a meta-analysis. *Am J Gastroenterol* 2008;103(9):2394–400.

306. Miller JP. Inflammatory bowel disease in pregnancy: a review. *J R Soc Med* 1986; 79:221–25.

307. Kane S, Kisiel J, Shih L, Hanauer S. HLA disparity determines disease activity through pregnancy in women with inflammatory bowel disease. *Am J Gastroenterol* 2004;99(8):1523–26.

308. Mahadevan U, Sandborn WJ, Li DK, et al. Pregnancy outcomes in women with inflammatory bowel disease: a large community-based study from Northern California. *Gastroenterology* 2007;133(4):1106–12.

309. Katz JA, Antoni C, Keenan GF, et al. Outcome of pregnancy in women receiving infliximab for the treatment of Crohn's disease and rheumatoid arthritis. *Am J Gastroenterol* 2004;99(12):2385–92.

310. Vasiliauskas EA, Church JA, Silverman N, et al. Case report: evidence for transplacental transfer of maternally administered infliximab to the newborn. *Clin Gastroenterol Hepatol* 2006;4(10):1255–58.

311. Cappell MS. The fetal safety and clinical efficacy of gastrointestinal endoscopy during pregnancy (Review). *Gastroenterol Clin North Am* 2003;32(1):123–79.

312. Christensen LA, Dahlerup JF, Nielsen MJ, et al. Azathioprine treatment during lactation. *Aliment Pharmacol Ther* 2008;28(10):1209–13.

313. Kane S, Ford J, Cohen R, Wagner C. Absence of infliximab in infants and breast milk from nursing mothers receiving therapy for Crohn's disease before and after delivery. *J Clin Gastroenterol* 2009;43(7):613–16.

Index